T0276187

Pediatric Electrocardiography

Ra-id Abdulla • William Bonney
Omar Khalid • Sawsan Awad
Editors

Pediatric Electrocardiography

An Algorithmic Approach to Interpretation

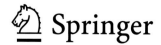

Springer

Editors
Ra-id Abdulla, MD
Department of Pediatric Cardiology
Rush University Medical Center
Chicago, IL, USA

William Bonney, MD
Department of Cardiology
Children's Hospital of Philadelphia
Philadelphia, PA, USA

Omar Khalid, MD
Department of Cardiology
Nationwide Children's Hospital
Columbus, OH, USA

Sawsan Awad, MD
Department of Pediatrics
Rush University Medical Center
Chicago, IL, USA

ISBN 978-3-319-26256-7   ISBN 978-3-319-26258-1   (eBook)
DOI 10.1007/978-3-319-26258-1

Library of Congress Control Number: 2016934595

Printed on acid-free paper

This Springer imprint is published by Springer Nature
The registered company is Springer International Publishing AG Switzerland

To our spouses, children, and families who define who we are.
And to our patients to whom we humbly offer our knowledge and efforts.

Ra-id Abdulla
William Bonney
Omar Khalid
Sawsan Awad

Preface

Like the heart itself, electrocardiograms (ECGs) wrap themselves with a shroud of mystery. With their squiggly lines and peaks and valleys that reflect the functions of the cardiac chambers that generate them, interpreting ECGs is perhaps the first attraction for young trainees to the field of cardiology. Daunting at first, but once the rules are learned, the hidden secrets of the heart become increasingly evident. It feels like detective's work, no clue is trivial, and the paradox can only be solved by the summation of all clues. However, it is this enigma that repels physicians in training and non-cardiologists from comprehending its benefits and reaping the most of its concealed information.

The ECG is frequently used as the first line of investigative studies when assessing a child with a symptom or sign suggesting a potential cardiac ailment. It is easy to order an ECG in the emergency room or in the outpatient office. The computerized interpretation provided in these settings is tempting to rely on, but unfortunately, it frequently leads to confusion as this particular interpretation tends to suggest pathology where none exists. All this culminates in supposition of cardiac disease, creating apprehension to patients and families and resulting in unwarranted referrals to pediatric cardiologists. This problem can be effectively averted once a reasonable level of proficiency in reading ECGs is attained through proper basic training, continued practice in reading ECGs, and having at hand a reference such as this book.

The first 4 chapters of this book discuss in details how electrical forces generated by the various cardiac chambers contribute to the normal ECG tracings. The subsequent 4 chapters review the various ECG abnormalities and the cardiac pathologies causing them. Chapter 9 details the various ECG presentations of systemic pathologies impacting the function and structure of the heart and as such resulting in aberrations of the ECG. Chapter 10 presents unique approach to ECG interpretation though algorithms. Throughout this book we have attempted to provide as many ECG illustrations and diagrams to make ECG learning effective.

Chapter 10 provides an analytical approach to electrocardiogram (ECG) reading through a practical approach of analyzing normal and abnormal findings of an ECG using a step by step methodological approach through algorithms. This process enables the formulation of competent differential diagnoses concisely and with ease when reviewing 12 lead ECGs and rhythm strips.

The illustrations used in this book are derived principally from electronically stored ECGs of patients that can be captured and reproduced for teaching purposes. In addition, many of the images presented were electronically drawn through computer programs allowing the production of clear and typical ECG findings.

Our hope in writing this book is to provide physicians, residents, students, and nurses with a concise reference for pediatric ECG and offer tools through which ECGs can be effectively and accurately read when performed in the inpatient or outpatient settings. Furthermore, we hope that our work will entice many young trainees to see the intrigue in electrocardiography and fall in love with this field, as we all did many years ago.

Chicago, IL, USA	Ra-id Abdulla, MD
Philadelphia, PA, USA	William Bonney, MD
Columbus, OH, USA	Omar Khalid, MD
Chicago, IL, USA	Sawsan Awad, MD

Contents

Contributors

Ra-id Abdulla, MD Pediatric Cardiology, Rush University Medical Center, Chicago, IL, USA

Maytham Al-kubaisi, MD Pediatric Cardiology, Rush University Medical Center, Chicago, IL, USA

Leen Alsaleh Pediatric Cardiology, Rush University Medical Center, Chicago, IL, USA

Sawsan Awad, MD Pediatric Cardiology, Rush University Medical Center, Chicago, IL, USA

William Bonney, MD Department of Cardiology, Children's Hospital of Philadelphia, Philadelphia, PA, USA

Jessica Bowman, MD Department of Pediatrics, The Ohio State University/Nationwide Children's Hospital, Columbus, OH, USA

Christopher Bugnitz, MD Department of Cardiology, Nationwide Children's Hospital, Columbus, OH, USA

Jessie Hu, MD Pediatric Cardiology, Rush University Medical Center, Chicago, IL, USA

Omar Jamil College of Medicine, University of Illinois Hospital, Chicago, IL, USA

Omar Khalid, MD Department of Cardiology, Nationwide Children's Hospital, Columbus, OH, USA

Kaitlin L'Italien, MD Department of Pediatric Cardiology, The Ohio State University/Nationwide Children's Hospital, Columbus, OH, USA

Carlos Miranda, MD Pediatric Cardiology, Rush University Medical Center, Chicago, IL, USA

Shaun Mohan, MD, MPH Department of Cardiology, Section of Electrophysiology, Texas Children's Hospital, Houston, TX, USA

Brieann Muller Pediatric Cardiology, Rush University Medical Center, Chicago, IL, USA

Cyndi Sosnowski, MD Pediatric Cardiology, Rush University Medical Center, Chicago, IL, USA

Anas Taqatqa, MD Pediatric Cardiology, Rush University Medical Center, Chicago, IL, USA

Carolyn M. Wilhelm, MD Department of Cardiology, Nationwide Children's Hospital, Columbus, OH, USA

The Normal Electrocardiogram

1

Carolyn M. Wilhelm and Omar Khalid

Developing a Systematic Approach

The electrocardiogram (ECG) is a graphical representation of the electrical activity of the heart. It is an important tool in the care of many patients with potential cardiovascular disease. Therefore, when approaching an ECG, it is essential to interpret each one in the same, systematic way in order to avoid missing important findings.

A typical approach to follow would include these steps:

1. Assess patient demographics (age, gender, and sex)
2. Standardization
3. Rate
4. Axis
   (a) P axis
   (b) QRS axis
   (c) T axis
5. Rhythm
6. AV conduction
   (a) P wave
   (b) PR interval
7. Ventricular conduction
   (a) QRS complex
   (b) QRS duration
   (c) ST segment and T wave
   (d) QT interval
   (e) JT Interval
   (f) U waves
8. Evaluation for chamber enlargement or hypertrophy

C.M. Wilhelm, MD • O. Khalid, MD (✉)
Department of Cardiology, Nationwide Children's Hospital,
700 Children's Drive, Columbus, OH 43204, USA
e-mail: Carolyn.wilhelm@nationwidechildrens.org;
Omar.Khalid@nationwidechildrens.org

Patient Demographics and Impact on Interpretation

Patient demographics are important to consider when interpreting ECGs, particularly in the pediatric population. Age, sex, race, and even body habitus can all have an effect on a patient's ECG.

Age

One must consider the patient's age during ECG interpretation as the normal values for the heart rate, measured intervals, axis, and voltage criteria are adjusted with age [see]. Heart rate is fastest at birth and then progressively decreases until the teenage years when patients reach their adult resting heart rate.

Davignon et al. published a study of 2,141 white Canadian children ages 0–16 years. The authors divided the patient population into 12 age groups to establish standard values for ECGs in normal children [1]. Similar trends have been noted in other recent studies [2–4]. The following observations were noted:

1. Heart rate – The mean heart rate increased from day one of life to the first month of age and then showed a slow decrease from 3 months of age on. The highest heart rate was recorded between 1 and 3 months of age with an average heart rate of 150 beats per minute.
2. QRS axis – QRS axis has been shown to vary with age as well, with the QRS axis for the first week of life on average being 135° and decreasing to 60° by 3–6 months of age.
3. P wave amplitude – The P wave amplitude in lead V2 shows a gradual decrease with age.
4. PR interval – The PR interval remains stable until approximately 3 months of age and then it gradually increases. The PR interval also increases as the heart rate decreases.

© Springer International Publishing Switzerland 2016
R. Abdulla et al. (eds.), *Pediatric Electrocardiography: An Algorithmic Approach to Interpretation*,
DOI 10.1007/978-3-319-26258-1_1

5. R and S wave amplitudes – R wave amplitude decreases with age in leads V3R and V1 and increases in lead V7, while the S wave shows an inverse trend. This leads to an overall steady decrease in the R/S ratio in leads V3R and V1 and increased R/S ratio in leads V6 and V7 with increased age.

6. QRS duration – The QRS duration increases with age and varies with heart rate.

7. Q wave amplitude – Maximum Q wave amplitudes are seen until age 1–3 years and then gradually decrease.

8. T wave changes – The T wave in leads VI and V3R is upright at birth. Between 3 and 7 days of life, the T wave becomes negative. The T wave will remain negative until 3–8 years of age when it becomes positive.

9. QTc interval – There is a small increase with age.

Body Habitus

Body habitus can have a major effect on QRS voltages. The adipose tissue can act as a form of insulation between the heart's electrical conduction and the ECG electrodes. With an increased distance from the heart to the ECG electrode, an ECG may appear to have lower overall voltage [5]. Studies performed in the adult population have shown that patients with hypertension and obesity could potentially not meet criteria for left ventricular hypertrophy (LVH) depending on the LVH criteria used for ECG interpretation [6, 7]. In 2012, Nasir et al. reported on 55,218 adult patients age 18–35 years and found that in patients with a BMI $\geq$18.5 kg/m^2, there was a decrease in R wave voltage as BMI increased and there was an increased R wave voltage with decreased BMI in patients with BMI <18.5 kg/m^2 [8].

Gender

Davignon et al. reported differences in ECG parameters found between males and females. A significant difference was noted in R wave amplitude between the sexes and suggested this value be stratified not only by age but also by sex [1]. Rijnbeek also documented a difference in Q, R, and S wave amplitudes showing that they were all significantly larger in males compared to females. It was also noted that the QRS duration is longer in males. On the other hand, the QTc (corrected QT interval) remained relatively stable across the age spectrum, but at approximately 15 years of age, normal females have a slightly longer QTc when compared to males [4].

Race

Normal values of QRS voltage can differ by race. In 1985, a study of 15–19-year-old children revealed that African American male patients have been shown to have a higher upper limit of normal QRS voltage compared to European-descended Americans [9]. In a separate study of North American white, black, and Hispanic patients, there was also a higher limit of normal QRS voltage for African American patients compared to white patients. This was seen in both men and women, but in women, it was only evident in women >34 years of age. In comparison to white patients, Hispanic men and women were noted to have a lower limit of normal for QRS voltage [10].

Standardization

The ECG signal is standardized so that 1 mV deflection is equal to 10 mm in height (full standardization). The standardization is marked at the beginning of the ECG with a calibration signal that produces a rectangle that is two big boxes tall (10 mm) and five small boxes wide (25 mm).

Occasionally when the voltages are high, the gain can be adjusted to "half standardization." In this setting, 1 mV = 1 big box (5 mm); therefore, the voltage complex has to be multiplied by two for calculations. On the other hand, "double standardization" can be set in cases where the voltages are too small, in this setting 1 mV = 4 big boxes (20 mm). In this case, the voltage complex has to be divided by two for calculations (Fig. 1.1).

Other modes of standardization are less frequently used (Fig. 1.2). In each case of standardization, calculation must take in consideration the type of standardization and the leads it affects. The examples shown in Fig. 1.2 suggest that not all leads are standardized equally and as such calculation of actual heights and depths of ECG waves must be corrected accordingly.

Rate and Rhythm

Rate

Each ECG is printed on gridded paper, which has a speed of 25 mm per second. Each small box is 1 mm and represents 0.04 s. Thus, each large box is 5 mm and 0.2 s (Fig. 1.3).

Rate is calculated by measuring either the P-P or R-R interval. The interval should be measured from the beginning of either the P wave or the QRS wave to the beginning of the next corresponding wave. Measuring from the peak of either wave can be inaccurate in patients with abnormal conduction (Fig. 1.4).

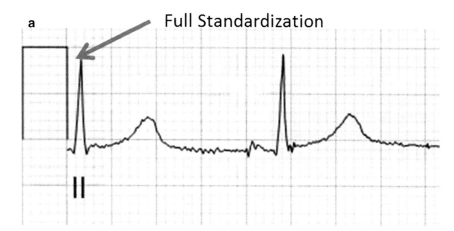

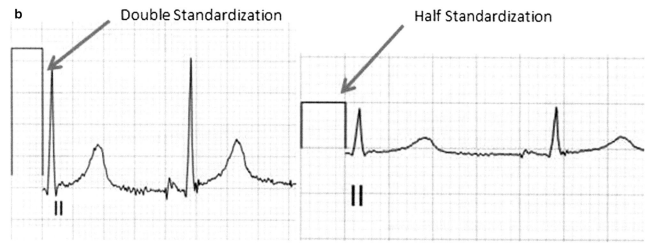

Fig. 1.1 Examples of common standardization. (**a**) Full standardization. (**b**) Examples of double standardization and half standardization

Fig. 1.2 Examples of less common standardization: (**a**) Limb leads normal standardization and precordial leads half standardization. (**b**) Precordial leads normal standardization and limb leads half standardization. (**c**) Limb leads normal standardization and precordial leads double standardization. (**d**) Precordial leads normal standardization and limb leads double standardization

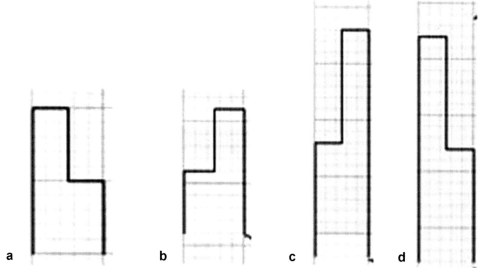

Lead II is typically used to calculate the rate. This lead is usually one of the leads used to record the rhythm strip located at the bottom of the ECG. A different lead can be considered if the tracing has fewer artifacts than lead II.

In order to estimate the heart rate quickly, several different techniques can be used:

1. For slower rates, the number of large boxes is divided by 300 (Fig. 1.5).

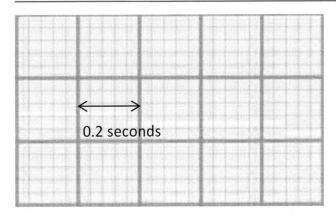

Fig. 1.3 Each large box (5 mm) on ECG grid paper is equivalent to 0.2 s

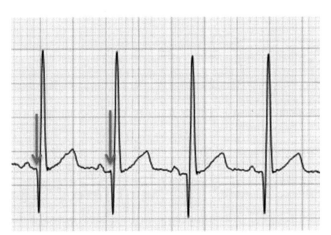

Fig. 1.4 Example ECG. The distance between the two large *arrows* is 11 small boxes or 0.44 s. To calculate beats per minute: 60/0.44 = 136 beats per minute

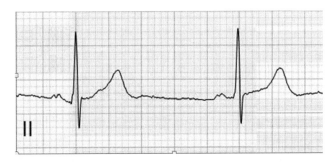

Fig. 1.5 Five large boxes between QRS's: 300/5 = 60. Estimated rate is 60 bpm

2. For faster heart rates, the number of QRS complexes is counted within six large boxes (1.2 ms) and multiplied by 50 (Fig. 1.6).
3. For rapid calculation, the number of large boxes between two consecutive R-R intervals is measured (Fig. 1.7):
   1. Box = 0.2 s 60/0.2 = 300 bpm
   2. Boxes = 0.4 s 60/0.4 = 150 bpm

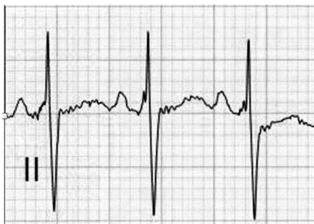

Fig. 1.6 Three QRS complexes within 6 large boxes: 50 × 3 = 150. Estimated rate 150 bpm

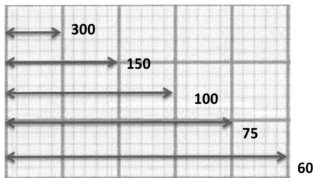

Fig. 1.7 Heart rate calculation can be quickly estimated by counting the number of large boxes between two consecutive R-R intervals. Heart rate is listed in beats per minute

   3. Boxes = 0.6 s 60/0.6 = 100 bpm
   4. Boxes = 0.8 s 60/0.8 = 75 bpm
   5. Boxes = 1 s 60/1 = 60 bpm

The heart rate is variable in the normal heart. It is regulated by both the parasympathetic and sympathetic nervous systems. Parasympathetic activity (vagal nerve stimulation) will lead to decreased heart rate, and sympathetic activity leads to an increased heart rate. At rest, parasympathetic input is higher and the heart rate will be lower. With activity, the sympathetic tone is higher and the heart rate will be increased [11].

The heart rate in the pediatric population varies with age (Appendix 1). In adults, tachycardia is defined as a heart rate greater than 100 bpm and bradycardia as less than 60 bpm. For children, this must be defined by a heart rate greater than the upper limit of normal (tachycardia) or less than the lower limit of normal (bradycardia).

Rhythm

The normal rhythm of the heart is called a sinus rhythm, in which, cardiac impulses originate from the sinoatrial (SA) node.

Criteria for sinus rhythm:

1. Normal P wave axis and morphology
2. A single P wave before every QRS
3. A single QRS following each P wave

Axis: P Wave, QRS, and T Wave

This section is further detailed in Chap. 3. ECG recordings can provide information about the direction and magnitude of various complexes. The electric axis (direction of the net electric force in the heart) can change in different cardiac conditions such as mechanical shifts, chamber enlargement or hypertrophy, or conduction disturbances.

In order to assess the axis on an ECG, knowledge of the normal vectoral forces of each lead is essential (Fig. 1.8).

P Wave Axis

The P axis is the mean vector of atrial depolarization. A normal P wave axis is one criterion for a sinus rhythm. A sinus P wave is an atrial depolarization originating from the sinoatrial node. The electrical activity generated is moving from the high right atrium to low septal right atrium and in general is moving from the right side of the heart to a leftward direc-

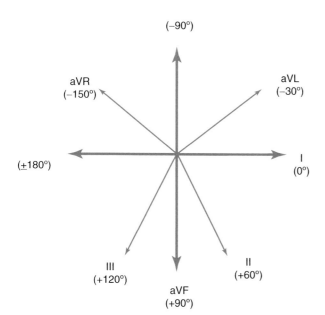

Fig. 1.8 Normal vectoral forces for each limb lead

tion. Based on this information, a sinus P wave will appear as a positive P wave in leads I, II, and aVF and negative in lead aVR. This generates an axis of 0 to +90° (Fig. 1.9).

QRS Axis

The QRS axis is the mean vector of ventricular depolarization. The dominating ventricular depolarization forces in the newborn are right-sided forces, and thus, the axis will be rightward in the normal newborn ECG. Over time, the forces of the heart become predominantly left sided and the axis will shift left compared to the newborn [1] (Appendix, Table 1). To determine QRS axis, leads I, II, and aVF are usually examined (Figs. 1.10 and 1.11).

T Wave Axis

The T wave axis is the mean vector of ventricular repolarization. The T wave axis is −40° to +100° between 0 and 7 days of life. By approximately 1 month of age, patients will reach the adult T wave axis of 0° to +90°. The QRS-T angle is the angle formed between the QRS axis and T wave axis. Abnormal QRS-T angle may occur in ventricular hypertrophy with strain or ventricular conduction abnormalities.

Abnormal T wave axis may be associated with:

1. Ventricular hypertrophy with strain
2. Myocarditis
3. Pericarditis
4. Myocardial ischemia
5. Bundle branch block

Atrioventricular (AV) Conduction

P Wave

The P wave represents atrial depolarization. It can take on different morphologies, but the typical P wave is characterized by a symmetric mound-shaped wave. Biphasic and notched P waves can also be seen in children. The duration of the P wave should be no longer than 0.08 s in children less than 12 months of age or 0.1 s in older children [12] (Fig. 1.12).

PR Interval

The conduction from the atria to ventricle is represented by the PR interval. As previously noted, the PR interval does change with age and heart rate (refer to PR intervals by age and heart rate in Appendix, Tables 1, 2). It is best assessed in

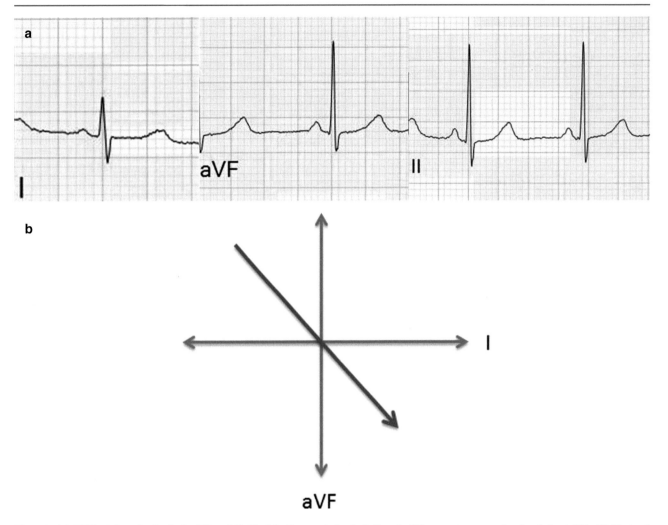

Fig. 1.9 (**a**) ECG tracings for leads I, aVF, and II. Upright P wave in leads I, II and aVF suggest a normal axis of about 60°. (**b**) Vectoral estimate

lead II. The PR interval is calculated by measuring from the beginning of the P wave to the first deflection of the QRS (negative deflection if a Q wave or positive if an R wave) (Fig. 1.13).

Interventricular Conduction

The QRS Complex

The QRS complex represents ventricular depolarization (Fig. 1.14).

- The *Q wave* is characterized by the first downward/negative deflection from the baseline.
- The *R wave* is an upward/positive inflection from the baseline.
- The *S wave* is a downward/negative deflection from the baseline that occurs after the R wave.

If there is an upward/positive deflection that occurs after the S wave, this is referred to as an R'. An R' can be found in approximately 5 % of the healthy population (Fig. 1.15).

Capitalized letters indicate a major deflection from the baseline, and lowercase letters indicate a minor deflection from the baseline. A deflection is considered minor if it is less than one-half the amplitude of a major deflection.

Q Waves

The Q wave represents the left to right depolarization of the ventricular septum. Although Q waves are considered an abnormal finding in the adult population, they can be a benign finding in the pediatric population. It is commonly seen in the inferior leads (II, III, aVF) and the lateral leads (I, V5, V6). To distinguish normal from abnormal Q waves, assess the amplitude and duration.

Normal Q waves are small and narrow. It is usually less than one small box (1 mm) wide and no more than two small

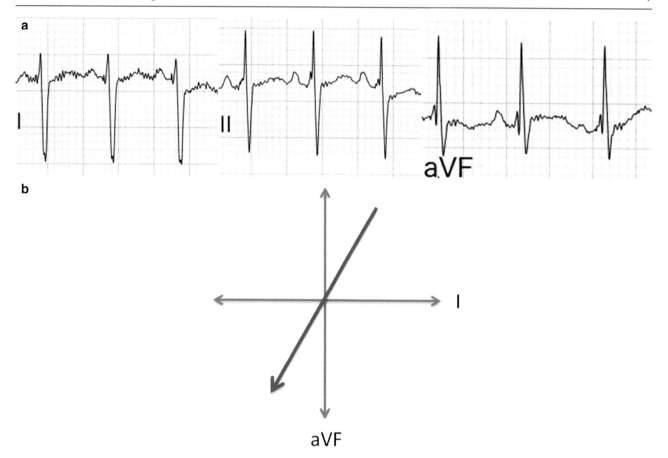

Fig. 1.10 (**a**) Leads I, II, and aVF from a 1-day-old patient. The net deflection in lead I is negative. The net deflection in lead II is negative. The net deflection in lead aVF is positive. (**b**) The overall vector is directed to a QRS axis of approximately 120° (+90° – +180°)

boxes (2 mm) deep, although leads III and aVR may have deeper Q waves that are still normal.

An important example to note of abnormal Q waves is the EKG finding of patients with anomalous left coronary artery from the pulmonary artery (ALCAPA). These patients will have deep, abnormal Q waves in leads I and aVL. This is an indication of left ventricular ischemia [13].

QRS Duration

The QRS duration is the time required for ventricular depolarization. It is measured from the beginning of the Q wave to the end of the S wave (Fig. 1.16). As previously noted, the QRS duration increases with age (due to the increase the ventricular muscle mass) and decreased heart rate. The QRS duration is best assessed in lead V5 (Appendix, Table 1).

R and S Wave Amplitude

R and S wave amplitude should be examined in each patient in order to determine if there is potential ventricular hypertrophy (Appendix 1).

ST Segment and T Waves

The ST segment represents the time between the S wave (end of ventricular depolarization) and T wave (ventricular repolarization). The ST segment is usually at the same level as the baseline (determined by the PR segment). It can be considered normal to have an upward slanting of the ST segment. This is commonly referred to as early repolarization (Fig. 1.17).

The T wave represents ventricular repolarization. It is usually asymmetric and has low amplitude. The T wave is best assessed in the lateral precordial leads (V4–V6). The amplitude does vary by age. The T wave in lead V1 will have a positive deflection in the newborn and become negative during the first week of life. It will remain negative until early adolescence where it may become positive again [1, 15].

A T wave is generally considered low voltage when it is less than 2 mm and high voltage if it is greater than 7 mm in a limb lead or 10 mm in a precordial lead [12] (Fig. 1.18).

QT Interval

The QT Interval represents the time of ventricular depolarization and repolarization. Abnormal QT interval has been associated with serious ventricular arrhythmias. It is measured as

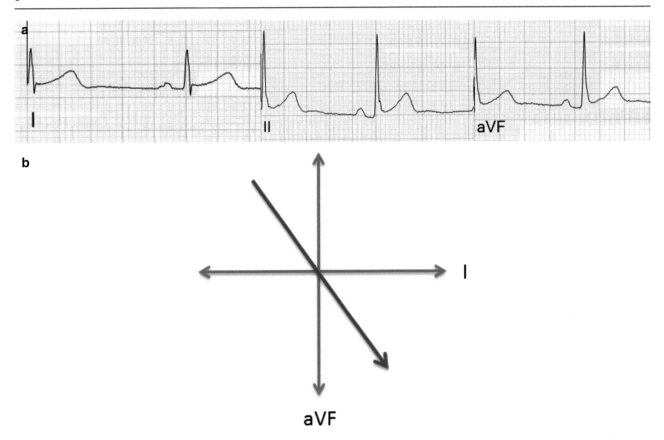

Fig. 1.11 (a) Leads I, II, and aVF from a 16-year-old patient. The net deflection in lead I is positive. The net deflection in lead II is positive. The net deflection in lead aVF is positive. (b) The overall vector is directed to a QRS axis of approximately 600 (00 - +900)

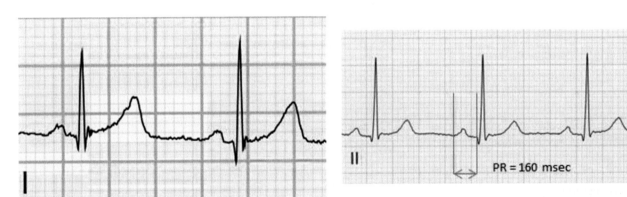

Fig. 1.12 Lead I of an ECG tracing demonstrating normal P waves

Fig. 1.13 ECG from a 16-year-old with a PR interval of 160 ms

the distance from the onset of the QRS complex to the end of the T wave. The QT interval is most accurately measured from leads II and V5. The QT interval varies with heart rate. This variation can be corrected by using the Bazett's formula [14].

$$QTc = \frac{QT\ intetval}{\sqrt{(RR\ interval)}}$$

The QTc is considered normal if it is <450 ms. In adolescent females, QTc is normal if it is <460 ms. There is currently no universally accepted lower limit for QTc. While there is a disease known as short QT syndrome, it is extremely rare and much less common than long QT syndrome. QTc measurements <330 for a male or <340 for a female would be concerning.

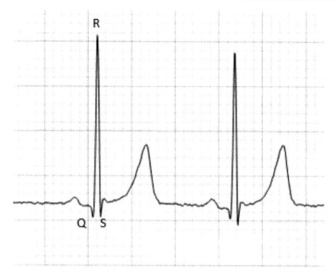

Fig. 1.14 ECG tracing of the QRS complex

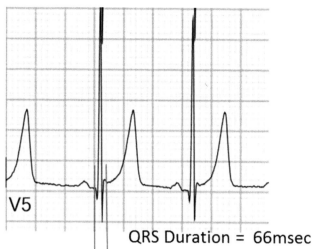

Fig. 1.16 Normal QRS duration of 66 ms in a 4-year-old child

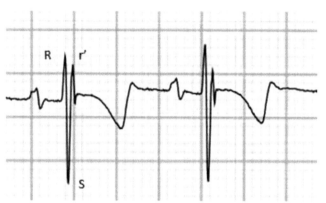

Fig. 1.15 ECG tracing demonstrating an RSr' pattern

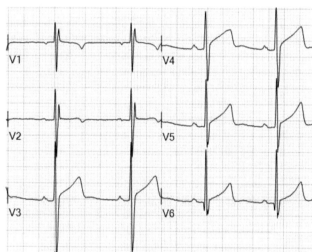

Fig. 1.17 ECG from a 17-year-old with early repolarization. Note the ST segment maintains an upward angle

JT Interval

In patients with ventricular conduction defects, the QT interval may be prolonged due to the long QRS duration (Fig. 1.19). Therefore, JT interval has been proposed as a more appropriate measure of ventricular repolarization than the QT. The JT interval represents the true ventricular repolarization. It is measured from the J point to the end of the T wave [16, 17].

Like the QT interval, the JT interval can also be corrected for rate using Bazett's formula. This will calculate a JTc.

$$JTc = \frac{JT\ intetval}{\sqrt{(RR\ interval)}}$$

U Waves

U waves are positive deflections found after the T wave and before the next atrial depolarization (P wave). The origin of this wave remains controversial. Normal U waves are less than one-half the amplitude of the T wave. They are more appreciated in the mid-precordial leads and in patients with slower heart rates. The ascent of the U wave is typically shorter than the descent [18, 19]. Normal U waves should not be included in the measurement of the QT interval (Fig. 1.20).

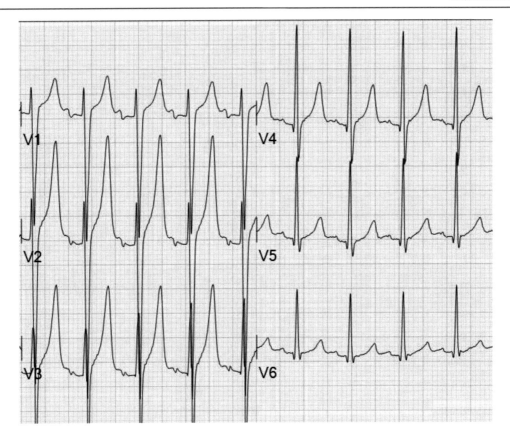

Fig. 1.18 Tall peaked T waves seen in the mid-precordial leads of a patient with diabetic ketoacidosis

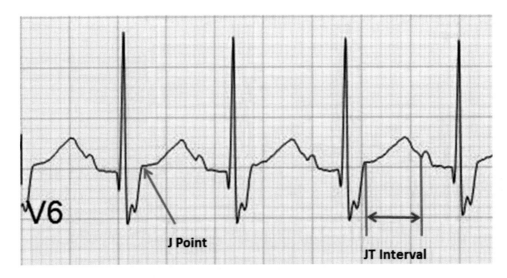

Fig. 1.19 ECG tracing demonstrating the location of the J point and JT interval

Fig. 1.20 ECG from a 16-year-old with no heart disease

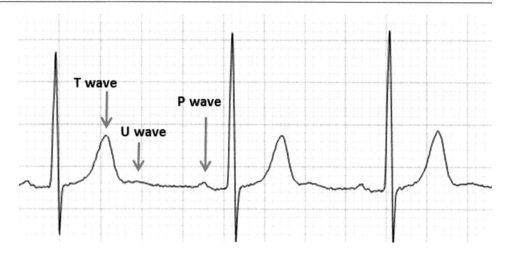

References

1. Davignon A, Rautaharju P, Boisselle E, et al. Normal ECG standards for infants and children. Pediatric Cardiol. (1979–1980);131:123–31.
2. Semizel E, Oztürk B, Bostan OM, et al. The effect of age and gender on the electrocardiogram in children. Cardiol Young. 2008;18(1):26–40.
3. Macfarlane PW, McLaughlin SC, Devine B, et al. Effects of age, sex, and race on ECG interval measurements. J Electrocardiol. 1994;27(Suppl):14–9.
4. Rijnbeek PR, Witsenburg M, Schrama E, et al. New normal limits for the paediatric electrocardiogram. Eur Heart J. 2001;22:702–11.
5. Hancock EW, Deal BJ, Mirvis DM, et al. AHA/ACCF/HRS recommendations for the standardization and interpretation of the electrocardiogram: part V: electrocardiogram changes associated with cardiac chamber hypertrophy: a scientific statement from the American Heart Association Electrocardiography and Arrhythmias Committee, Council on Clinical Cardiology; the American College of Cardiology Foundation; and the Heart Rhythm Society: endorsed by the International Society for Comperturized Electrocardiography. Circulation. 2009;119:e251–61.
6. Okin PM, Jern S, Devereux RB, et al. Effect of obesity on electrocardiographic left ventricular hypertrophy in hypertensive patients: the Losartan Intervention For Endpoint (LIFE) Reduction in Hypertension Study. Hypertension. 2000;35(1):13–8.
7. Abergel E, Tase M, Menard J, et al. Influence of obesity on the diagnostic value of electrocardiographic criteria for detecting left ventricular hypertrophy. Am J Cardiol. 1996;77(9):739–44.
8. Nasir JM, Rubal BJ, Jones SO, et al. The effects of body mass index on surface electrocardiograms in young adults. J Electrocardiol. 2012;45(6):646–51.
9. Rao PS. Racial differences in electrocardiograms and vectorcardiograms between black and white adolescents. J Electrocardiol. 1985;18(4):309–13.
10. Rautaharju PM, Zhou SH, Calhoun HP. Ethnic differences in ECG amplitudes in north american white, black, and Hispanic men and women. Effect of Obesity and Age. J Electrocardiol. 1994;27:20–31.
11. Shaffer F, McCraty R, Zerr CL. A healthy heart is not a metronome: an integrative review of the heart' s anatomy and heart rate variability. Front Psychol. 2014;5:1–19.
12. Garson A. The electrocardiogram in infants and children: a systematic approach. Philadelphia: Pennsylvania; 1983.
13. Shapiro J, Boxer R, Krongrad E. Echocardiography in infants with anomalous origin of the left coronary ARtery. Pediatr Cardiol. 1979;28:23–8.
14. Rautaharju PM, Surawicz B, Gettes LS. AHA/ACCF/HRS recommendations for the standardization and interpretation of the electrocardiogram: part IV: the ST segment, T and U waves, and the QT interval: a scientific statement from the American Heart Association Electrocardiography and Arrhythmias Committee, Council on Clinical Cardiology; the American College of Cardiology Foundatiion; and the Heart Rhythm Society: endorsed by the International Society for Comperturized Electrocardiography. Circulation. 2009;119:e241–50.
15. Dickinson DF. The normal ECG in childhood and adolescence. Heart. 2005;91(12):1626–30.
16. Rautaharju PM, Zhang ZM, Prineas R, et al. Assessment of prolonged QT and JT intervals in ventricular conduction defects. Am J Cardiol. 2004;93(3):1017–21.
17. Chiladakis J, Kalogeropoulos A, Koutsogiannis N, et al. Optimal QT/JT interval assessment in patients with complete bundle branch block. Ann Noninvasive Electrocardiol. 2012;17:268–76.
18. Surawicz B. U wave: facts, hypotheses, misconceptions, and misnomers. J Cardiovasc Electrophysiol. 1998;9:1117–28.
19. Eyer K. Support for a mechanico-electrical source of the "U" wave. J Electrocardiol. 2015;48(1):31–2.

Cellular Electrophysiology and Electrocardiography

2

Carlos Miranda, Anas Taqatqa, Cyndi Sosnowski,
Leen Alsaleh, and Ra-id Abdulla

Introduction

The heartbeat is a biological process, which consists of an electrical phenomenon essential to the cardiac cycle. Knowledge of the physiology of the cardiac action potential and its effects on the heart provides valuable information to help understand a wide range of cardiac pathologies and its manifestation through the electrocardiogram. The basic principles of normal cellular electrophysiology changes and its relationship to electrocardiography are reviewed in this chapter.

Cardiac Action Potential

Cardiac cells, like many other cells, are characterized by an electrical potential across the cell membrane. This action potential varies in a cyclical fashion in response to change in various electrolytes across the cell membrane. This variation in electrical potential occurs in stages (called phases) within each cardiac cycle [1, 2] (Fig. 2.1). The surface electrocardiogram represents the net action potentials of cardiac cells [3]. Cardiac cells possess one of two different patterns of action potential phases: fast response and slow response (Figs. 2.2a, b). The difference is mainly in the upstroke velocity at the start of depolarization.

C. Miranda, MD • A. Taqatqa, MD • C. Sosnowski, MD
R. Abdulla, MD (✉)
Pediatric Cardiology, Rush University Medical
Center, Chicago, IL, USA
e-mail: Carlos_D_Miranda@rush.edu; Anas_Taqtqa@rush.edu;
Cyndi_R_Sosnowski@rush.edu; rabdulla@rush.edu

L. Alsaleh
Pediatric Cardiology, Rush University Medical Center,
1650 W. Harrison Street, Chicago, IL 60612, USA

The Cardiac Cycle

Electrical events in cardiac cells eventually precipitate mechanical changes manifesting as atrial and ventricular contractions. Electrical stimulation of the heart starts at the sinoatrial (SA) node which excites the right atrium (RA). This impulse results in atrial depolarization which is represented by the P wave on the electrocardiogram (ECG). Atrial depolarization initiates contraction, or systole of the right and left atria. Atrial systole lasts for approximately 60 msec and is represented by the P–Q segment on the ECG. During the first 20 msec of atrial depolarization, the electrical changes of depolarization have already conducted halfway through the atria as represented by the P wave with an anterior, leftward and inferior axis (60°). The atria repolarize resulting in relaxation of the atrial walls and remains in diastole for the rest of the cycle. Atrial repolarization (Ta wave) is masked on the ECG by the QRS complex. Near the end of the atrial systole, impulses from the SA node reach the atrioventricular (AV) node through the internal pathways in the RA. The impulse then travels through the bundle of His and down the bundle branches. The His and bundle branches are fibers specialized for rapid transmission of electrical impulses on either side of the interventricular septum which leads to depolarization of both the right ventricle (right bundle branch) and left ventricle (left bundle branch). Both bundles terminate in the Purkinje fibers. The culmination of this pathway results in ventricular depolarization, which is represented by the QRS complex on the ECG. In ventricular systole (contraction), increased pressure in the ventricles forces the AV valves close. Ventricular pressures increase until they are higher than those in the pulmonary artery and aorta, at this point pulmonary and aortic valves open and blood is ejected from the ventricles. Ventricular systole occurs during the S–T segment on ECG. This is followed by relaxation of the ventricles (repolarization) which is represented by the T wave on ECG.

Fig. 2.1 Action potential and the corresponding surface ECG depolarization/repolarization. The electrolytes primarily responsible for each phase of action potential are indicated for each phase

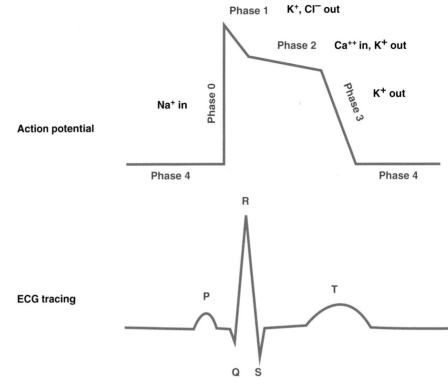

Action potential

ECG tracing

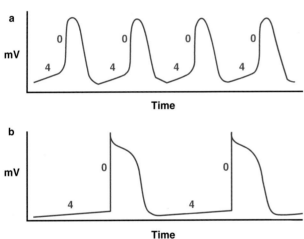

Fig. 2.2 (**a**, **b**) Diagrammatic comparison between (**a**) slow response cell (e.g., sinus node) and (**b**) fast response cell (e.g., Purkinje cell)

Resting Membrane Potential

The resting cardiac myocytes maintain a negative charge relative to the outside of the cell. Each cardiac myocyte has a membrane called the sarcolemma consisting of a lipid bilayer which prevents free exchange of intracellular-extracellular ions. Exchange of ions is possible through ion channels, ion pumps, and exchangers. Ion channels are narrow water-filled tunnels with selective permeability along with a gating mechanism to open and close the channel, which may be in

response to chemical or electrical signals, temperature, or mechanical forces [6]. Pumps, on the other hand, use energy to slowly move ions in order to maintain a gradient. The most important pump in establishing the resting membrane potential is the sodium-potassium ($Na^+–K^+$) ATPase pump. Through this pump, three sodium ions (Na^+) are pumped out of the cell in exchange for with two potassium ions (K^+) resulting in a resting membrane potential ranging from −80 to −90 mV. The sarcolemmal membrane along with its ion pumps and exchangers is a dynamic structure with changing permeability to various ions resulting in change in membrane potential at different points of the action potential (Fig. 2.3).

Sodium Channel

Sodium channels in myocytes are responsible for the rising phase (phase 0) of the action potentials. The rapid opening and closure of sodium channels lead to rapid depolarization of the sarcolemmal membrane and subsequently rapid conduction of the electrical signal. Stimulation by an action potential opens the sodium channel, allowing a small but significant number of Na + ions to move into the cell according to their electrochemical gradient, which results in further depolarization and changes the membrane potential toward sodium equilibration potential +40mv.

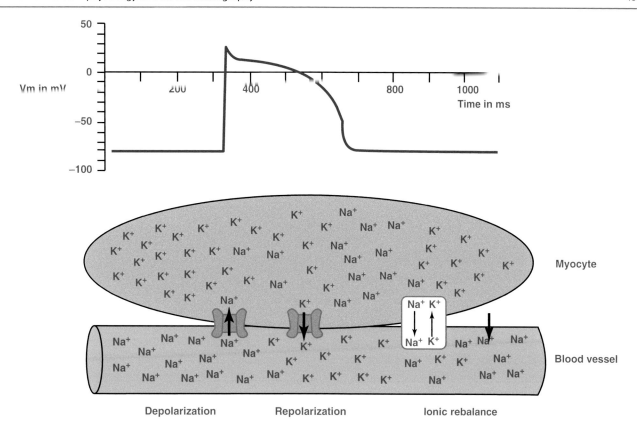

Fig. 2.3 This diagram represents electrical activation of a myocyte. Depolarization occurs secondary to rapid influx of sodium ions across the cell membrane. A plateau phase follows cardiac depolarization, and thereafter repolarization takes place. Repolarization is a consequence of the outflow of potassium ions

Potassium Channel

Potassium channels help to establish the resting membrane potential (phase 4), automaticity, the plateau phase (phase 2) of action potential, and repolarization.

1. The *transient outward current* (Ito) is voltage-gated and is activated without a delay. It is responsible for the early repolarization, creating "spike and dome" appearance of action potential in the ventricular myocyte. This current can be divided into two components:
   - Ca dependent and 4-aminopyridne insensitive carried by Cl- ions
   - Ca independent and 4-aminopyridine sensitive carried by K+ ions
   The density of *Ito* is variable, being greater in atrium than ventricle, greater in right ventricle than left ventricle, and greater in epicardium than endocardium.
2. The *delayed rectifier current* (Ik) is responsible for repolarization represented by phase 3 of action potential in myocytes. This current is activated as the membrane potential becomes more positive than −40 mV, producing outward currents that repolarize the cell. The expression of Ik is greater in the atrium than in the ventricles, which

explains the shorter action potential in atrial myocyte compared to ventricular myocyte. This channel can be divided into two components:
   - *Rapidly activating portion (Ikr):* Can be blocked by type 3 antiarrhythmic agent sotalol and its analogues. Other drugs that prolong action potential duration by affecting QT interval almost exclusively work on Ikr to produce their effect. Ikr gene (KCNH2) (HERG) is located on chromosome 7; abnormalities of this gene result in long QT syndrome.
   - *Slowly activating portion:* Becomes the dominant repolarizing current at more rapid heart rates. It is not affected by antiarrhythmic type 3. The gene for this channel is located on chromosome 11 and its abnormalities result in long QT syndrome type 1. Recently, there has been a third component described: ultra rapid delayed rectifier current, which has very rapid activation kinetics, and slow inactivation current. It is more sensitive to potassium channel blockers (type 3 antiarrhythmic), and its gene is located on chromosome 12.
3. *Inwardly rectifying currents*: (IK-ATP, Ik1, Ik-Ach)
   (IK-ATP): or ATP-sensitive potassium channels, which is activated when there is a drop in ATP levels (ischemia)

(Ik1): is responsible for stabilizing the resting membrane potential, shaping the initial depolarization, and final repolarization of the action potential.

(Ik-Ach): is activated by the binding of acetylcholine to the muscarinic receptor on the sarcolemmal membrane, localized primarily in nodal cells and atrial myocytes. Activation of the channels causes hyperpolarization of nodal cells and a slowing of the rate of spontaneous depolarization and shortening of the action potential in atrial and ventricular myocytes.

Calcium Channel

Calcium channels have several calcium binding sites; when these sites are devoid of calcium, the channel passes sodium ions freely. There are two main types of these channels:

1. *The L-type calcium channel (Ica,L long acting)*: activates at a more positive membrane potential (strong depolarization) and inactivates slowly. This type of channels serves for calcium inward current into the myocyte during plateau phase which triggers calcium-dependent calcium release from the sarcoplasmic reticulum.
2. *The T-type calcium channel (Ica,T transient)*: This channel activates at weak depolarization and inactivates rapidly. ICa-T is relatively insensitive to dihydropyridines or cadmium but is blocked by nickel. This type is most prominent in nodal cells where it is crucial for depolarization.

Gap Junctions

Gap junctions are small protein tubular structures that allow free movement of ions from the interior of one cell to the interior of the next. Each of these is composed of two connexons (or hemichannels), which connect across the intercellular space. These channels allow action potentials to travel easily from one cardiac muscle cell to the next. The connexon is composed of six connexin subunits, each of which has four transmembrane-spanning domains and two extracellular loops. The transmembrane domains and extracellular loops in all of the connexins are highly preserved while the intracellular loop between the second and third domain and the carboxy-terminus are highly variable which explains the difference in junction conductance, pH dependence, voltage dependence, and selectivity.

Types and Phases of Action Potential

The action potential of a cardiac myocyte results from a complex series of transmembrane ion fluxes. The main ions essential for this task include sodium, potassium, and calcium

ions, which create an electrical current through the cell membrane. Cardiac cells are of two types when considering action potential; these are:

1. *Fast response action potential:* this is noted in myocardial cells of the atria, ventricles, and His-Purkinje system [2, 3]. At the resting stage, these cells are negatively charged where the cell interior is negative with respect to the exterior. The negative resting potential is the result of potassium ions influx into the cells and the relative impermeability to sodium ions [7]. This is called the resting membrane potential where the magnitude is around −90 mV. Fast response action potential cells go through the following five phases during the cardiac cycle (Figs. 2.2 and 2.4):

Phase 4 (Resting Membrane Potential): The non-nodal cardiac cell's resting potential remains constant throughout the diastolic interval. The inward-rectifier current (IK1) remains the dominant conductance at rest and it is largely responsible for setting the resting membrane potential (about −90 mv). Other ATP-dependent pumps including the Na+−K ion exchange pump, Na+−Ca2+ exchanger current, and the Ik1 current also help maintain this electrical gradient. Slow depolarization which allows the membrane potential to increase due to a potassium efflux and a net sodium influx. This will continue until an electrical stimulus is received from the sinoatrial (SA) node, which would induce rapid depolarization at around −65 m. A lack of an SA node signal could allow the membrane potential to reach a threshold potential (pacemaker potential) of about −40 mV. This specific type of depolarization is known as automaticity where essentially the cells will depolarize taking over as the pacemaker [4].

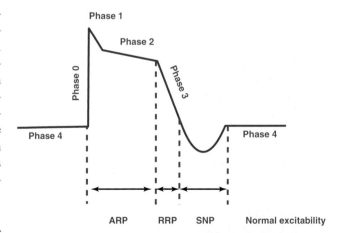

Fig. 2.4 Diagrammatic representation of a fast response action potential showing the time course of refractoriness and excitability. *ARP* absolute refractory period, *RRP* relative refractory period, *SNP* supernormal period. During phase 3 there is the absolute refractory period (*ARP*). If a strong enough stimulus occurs during this phase, another depolarization can occur given the ARP has passed

Phase 0 (Action Potential Upstroke): Before reaching phase 0, the resting membrane potential in phase 4 is about −90 mV. Potassium channels provide the dominant membrane conductance at rest until membrane potential reaches approximately −65 mV, which is the threshold level when sodium channels open. After electrical stimulation typically by a current from an adjacent cell through a gap junction, the cell membrane becomes mostly permeable to sodium instead of potassium resulting in an influx of Na ions. The difference in the extracellular sodium concentration of about 140 mM when compared to the intracellular concentration of about 4 mM drives the inward influx of Na. This causes a less negative membrane potential which represents depolarization of the upstroke of phase 0. The membrane potential does not quite reach the sodium equilibrium potential of approximately +40 mV, but stops at approximately +25 mV and then starts to repolarize. Phase 0 is the most rapid phase taking only several milliseconds to complete. The speed of phase 0 is governed by the change in voltage over the change in time and is known as the Vmax.

Phase 1 (Initial Repolarization): Inactivation of the sodium channels essentially terminates the action potential upstroke. This is followed by a negative deflection of the action potential, which is primarily due to the efflux of potassium through the cardiac transient outward potassium current (Ito). The outward flow of these positively charged ions results in a decrease of the transmembrane voltage or repolarization. The Ito current is then quickly deactivated which ends phase 1 of the action potential.

Phase 2 (Plateau): Before further repolarization, there is a delay or plateau that occurs. There is influx of calcium through the L-type calcium channels, which is balanced by an efflux of potassium through the Ik current. This large influx of calcium initiates the contraction of those cells throughout the plateau phase.

Phase 3 (Rapid Repolarization): The inactivation of L-type calcium channels marks the end of the plateau phase. The potassium channels remain open to allow for an increased leak and therefore a negative change in membrane potential (about −90 mV). However, a second depolarization can also occur during phase 3 of fast response action potential after the absolute refractory period has passed. This is called spontaneous depolarization or pacemaker potential. In this phase, it is possible to re-excite myocardial cells if enough time has elapsed since the initial repolarization from phase 0 and the absolute voltage of the cell membrane have been reattained. Usually in a Purkinje cell about 200 ms must pass since phase 0 and the membrane potential must return to about −55 mV. Sodium is also responsible for this type of depolarization as long as the refractory period has passed and stronger-than-usual stimulus is present [5].

2. Slow response action potential is characteristic of sino-atrial (SA) node and atrioventricular (AV) node cells. This type of action potential is different from the fast response action potential in the following ways [2, 8–10]:

(a) The resting potential is around −60 mV in comparison to the fast response resting potential which is lower at around −90 mV.

(b) The upstroke velocity at the start of depolarization is not as high, resulting in slower cell conduction velocity.

(c) Depolarization is a consequence of the slow influx of calcium and sodium ions, whereas the fast response action potential is dependent upon the fast sodium influx; this allows the automaticity of these cells.

Cardiac pacemaker cells' action potential is of the slow type. Unlike the cardiac myocytes, a pacemaker cell does not require stimulation to initiate their action potential. These cells undergo spontaneous depolarization and an action potential is triggered when threshold voltage is reached. Pacemaker cells have an unstable membrane potential and have fewer inward-rectifier K+ channels than do the cardiomyocytes so their transmembrane potential (TMP) is never lower then −60 mV. Also, there is no rapid depolarization phase as in cardiac myocytes and as such there is no need for a TMP of −90 mV to reconfigure into an active state. Cardiac cells that can display pacemaker behavior are primarily the SA node and secondarily the AV node and bundle of His. Once the threshold of −40 to −30 mV is reached in these pacemaker cells, an action potential is triggered. Phase 0 (upstroke) of the action potential, which depends on the activation of the L-type calcium channels, results in reversal of the membrane potential to a peak of about +10 mV. This increasing in the membrane potential leads to the opening of the potassium channels, which results in repolarization or phase 3 toward the resting membrane potential of −60 to −70 mV or phase 4 at which point the cycle is spontaneously repeated.

Currents responsible for automaticity include the slow sodium channels, which activate when the TMP is less than −55 mV. Inward sodium current is through the funny channels (If) and causes a slow depolarization. These channels are turned on by repolarization from the proceeding action potential. Once this slow action potential reaches −55 mV, T-type Ca2+ channels open for continued slow depolarization. Once TMP is between −40 and −30 mV, the threshold potential is reached for the pacemaker cells and the L-type Ca2+ channels open to depolarize the cells to +40 mV. Delayed rectifier potassium channels counterbalance the calcium channels which results in a plateau phase and then a return of the TMP back to −60 mV as the calcium channels close.

The Dipole Concept

When thinking about depolarization, it is important to remember that the current flow acts like a dipole. A dipole is when there is a single positive and negative charge close to one another. In cardiac cells, the negative charge is on the inside and the positive charge is on the outside. When there is a stimulus and sodium rushes into the cell during depolarization, the current also stimulates nearby areas of the cell membrane to do the same. Therefore depolarization produces a dipole and the current through the heart to producing a series of dipoles. The dipole then creates a vector by which the direction of current travels and propagates throughout the cardiac cells to cause contraction [5].

Refractory Period

The refractory period is essentially the period during which the pacemaker cells cannot evoke another action potential. It allows for relaxation of cardiac muscles and filling of the heart chambers. The refractory period has two components: absolute refractory, during which no action potential can be induced, and relative refractory during which action potential can be induced in response to supernormal stimulus. Depolarization must spread through the muscle to initiate the chemical processes that causes contraction.

The ventricles remain contracted until after repolarization has occurred, that is, until after the end of the T wave. The atria repolarize about 0.15–0.20 s after termination of the P wave, which is approximately when the QRS complex is being recorded in the electrocardiogram

References

1. Barry DM, Nerbonne JM. Myocardial potassium channels: electrophysiological and molecular diversity. Annu Rev Physiol. 1996;58:363–94.
2. Roden DM, George AL. Structure and function of cardiac sodium and potassium channels. Am J Physiol. 1997;273:H511–25.
3. Cranefield PF, Klein HO, Hoffman BF. Conduction of the cardiac impulse. 1. Delay, block, and one-way block in depressed Purkinje fibers. Circ Res. 1971;28(2):199–219.
4. Costanzo L. Physiology. 3rd ed. Philadelphia: Saunders Elsevier; 2006. p. 126–31.
5. Garson A. The electrocardiogram in infants and children: a systematic approach. Philadelphia: Lea & Febiger; 1983. p. 9–16.
6. MacDonald DI. Clinical cardiac electrophysiology in the young. New York: Springer; 2006. p. 17–31.
7. Snyders DJ. Structure and function of cardiac potassium channels. Cardiovasc Res. 1999;42:377–90.
8. Hille B. Ion channels of excitable membranes. Sunderland: Sinauer; 2001.
9. Roden DM, Balser JR, Geroge AL, Anderson ME. Cardiac ion channels. Annu Rev Physiol. 2002;64:431–75.
10. Grant AO. Cardiac ion channels. Circ Arrhythm Electrophysiol. 2009;2(2):185–94.

Cardiac Axis: Calculation and Interpretation

3

Anas Taqatqa, Brieann Muller, Maytham Al-kubaisi, Omar Jamil, Sawsan Awad, and Ra-id Abdulla

Mean Vector (Axis)
Introduction

During a cardiac cycle, the vectors of cardiac forces change in both direction and magnitude. The mean vector, which is the average of the direction and magnitude of the various vectors that exist in any instant at any point in the cardiac cycle, can be calculated using a 12-lead ECG. Abnormal axis can indicate aberrant heart structure, chamber hypertrophy/hypoplasia, or abnormal electrical conduction. The mean vector demonstrate the general direction of depolarization. The "axis" used to determine the position of the vector is centered at the AV node. The P wave, QRS complex, and T wave are the most commonly calculated mean vectors due to their clinical relevance [1].

Electrical forces generated by the cardiac chambers as they depolarize can be detected by the ECG limb leads. Any depolarization force traveling toward a particular lead will register as a positive deflection, while forces traveling away from a lead register as a negative deflection. Limb leads (I, II, III, aVR, aVL, and aVF) provide a precise methodology of determining the depolarization of the various cardiac axes.

The summation of electrical forces traveling through cardiac structures produces a mean vector of electrical force. The spatial direction of these mean vectors can be determined through ECG leads. For example, atrial depolarization initiated at the sinus node, located in the high right atrium, spreads down the right atrium as well as leftward toward the left atrium to terminate at the AV node. These electrical changes have a mean vector which is mostly leftward and inferior as detected by the limb leads, therefore registering as a positive deflection in all the inferior and leftward leads (I, II, III, and aVF) and negative in aVR.

P-Wave Mean Vector

P-wave axis determines the origin of the pacemaker impulse for the cardiac rhythm. P wave is the result of depolarization from the sinus node to the AV node. In a normal sinus rhythm, the atrial depolarization originates from the sinus node located at the high right atrium at the superior vena cava-right atrial junction. Depolarization travels from that point inferiorly and leftward toward the AV node. Therefore, a normal P-wave axis is somewhere between 0 and 90°. Typically, P-wave axis is about 60°, similar to Lead II. As such P wave appears most prominent in this lead, rendering this lead most suitable for use with cardiac monitors.

Abnormal P-wave axis suggests that the cardiac pacemaker is not the sinus node, or in rare cases, the sinus node is located in an abnormal position, such as in a left-sided atrium as in situs inversus. Pacemaker activity induced by the right or left atria tissue will also cause abnormal depolarization [2] (Table 3.1).

A. Taqatqa, MD • B. Muller • M. Al-kubaisi, MD
R. Abdulla, MD (✉)
Pediatric Cardiology, Rush University Medical Center,
Chicago, IL, USA
e-mail: Anas_Taqtqa@rush.edu; brieann_a_muller@rush.edu;
Maytham_A_Al-kubaisi@rush.edu; rabdulla@rush.edu

O. Jamil
College of Medicine, University of Illinois Hospital,
808 S Wood St, Chicago, IL 60612, USA
e-mail: janil2@uic.edu

S. Awad, MD
Pediatric Cardiology, Rush University
Medical Center, 1650 W. Harrison Street,
Chicago, IL 60612, USA
e-mail: Sawsan_M_Awad@rush.edu

© Springer International Publishing Switzerland 2016
R. Abdulla et al. (eds.), *Pediatric Electrocardiography: An Algorithmic Approach to Interpretation*,
DOI 10.1007/978-3-319-26258-1_3

Table 3.1 Interpretation of P wave axis

P-wave axis	Origin of pacemaker	Potential causes
0–90°	Sinus node	Normal pattern
	Ectopic high right atrium	Ectopic atrial pacemaker
	Right atrium	Electronic atrial pacemaker
90–180°	Sinus node in normal position with erroneous ECG data	Wrong lead connection (placing right limb leads on left limbs and vice versa)
	Sinus node in high left-sided atrium	Heterotaxy
180–270°	Ectopic low left atrium	Ectopic atrial pacemaker
270–0°	Ectopic low right atrium	Ectopic atrial pacemaker

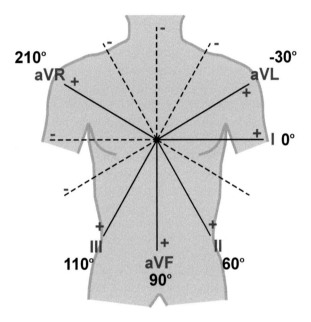

Fig. 3.1 Limb leads are leads: I, II, III, aVR, aVL, and aVF. Leads I and aVF are perpendicular to each other; using these two leads allows easy assessment of QRS axis. Lead I is at 0°, Lead II is at 60°, Lead aVF is at 90°, Lead III is at 110°, Lead aVR is at 210°, Lead aVL is at −30°

QRS Mean Vector (Axis)

The QRS mean vector is an important calculation when reading an ECG as it provides vital information regarding ventricular depolarization, conduction abnormalities, chamber hypertrophy, and other crucial data. As with the P wave, this axis is determined by the frontal plane leads [3].

The QRS mean vector between 0 and 7 days is about +135° and progressively decreases to about +60° in the age range of 3–6 months and remains stable after this age [5]. The range for the axis in the first month of a full-term neonate is +55 to +200° (Figs. 3.3 and 3.4), while the range for a premature neonate is +65 to +174°, more to the left. [4]

Lead I and aVF are perpendicular to each other and are the easiest to use when determining the QRS axis. In younger patients, aVR and Lead III may be incorporated in this process. Lead I represents a horizontal line, while Lead aVF is a vertical line perpendicular to Lead I and crossing it in a "plus"-sign fashion (Figs. 3.1 and 3.2).

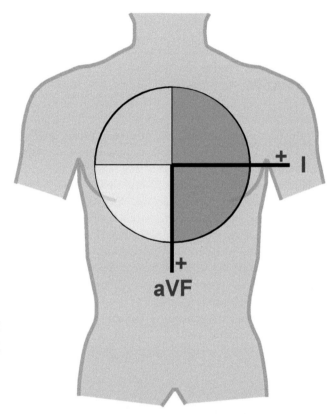

Fig. 3.2 Leads I and aVF are perpendicular to each other and divide the axis wheel into four quadrants. In this diagram green represents southeast, normal quadrant for P and RQS axes for all ages. Yellow is southwest quadrant, a normal region for QRS axis in infants and young children. Beige is northwest quadrant, QRS axis in this quadrant represents right axis deviation for all age groups. The blue quadrant is northeast quadrant where P and QRS axes in this quadrant are normal in adults if 0°–30°; otherwise it represents left axis deviation for QRS axis

There are different methods used in estimating the QRS mean vector; these include:

Quadrant-Based QRS Axis Determination

This provides a rough idea of the general direction of the QRS mean vector; although not precise, it most of the times suffices (Figs. 3.2 and 3.3).

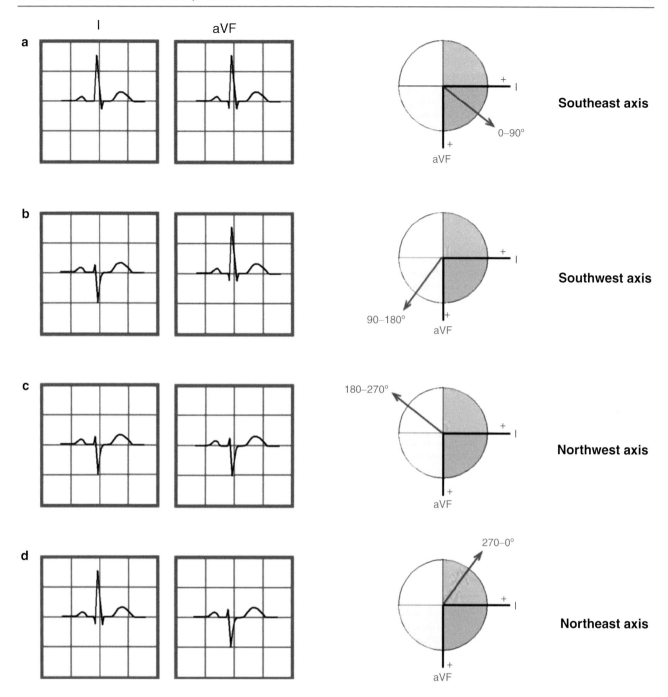

Fig. 3.3 Various combinations of QRS complexes in Leads I and aVF and the resulting axes: (**a**) QRS is net positive in Leads I and aVF. QRS axis is southwest (0–90°). (**b**) QRS is net negative in Lead I and positive in Lead aVF. QRS axis is southeast (90–180°). (**c**) QRS is net negative in Leads I and aVF. QRS axis is northwest (180–270°). (**d**) QRS is net positive in Lead I and negative in Lead aVF. QRS axis is northeast (270–0°)

Determine if the QRS complexes in Leads I and aVF are mostly positive or negative. If QRS complex is mostly positive in Lead I, then the QRS axis has an eastward direction; if negative it has a westward direction. In addition, if the QRS complex is mostly positive in Lead aVF, then the QRS complex has a southward direction, and if the QRS complex is mostly negative in Lead aVF, then it has a northward direction. By overlapping these two observations, you are left with a vector axis heading in one of the four quadrant direction:

Southeast: 0–90
Southwest: 90–180
Northwest: 180–270
Northeast: 270–0

The Neutral (Isoelectric) QRS Method

If positive and negative deflections are equal, this suggests a neutral summation (isoelectric), and when observed in one lead, then the axis of the QRS is perpendicular to that lead. For example, a neutral deflection in Lead aVF means that the QRS axis is either 90° if the QRS defection is mostly positive in Lead I (Fig. 3.4a) or 270° if the dominant deflection in I is negative (Fig. 3.4b).

This method quickly approximates the QRS mean vector and determines whether or not it is within the normal range or if the QRS mean vector has a right or left axis deviation.

Similarly, if the most isoelectric lead is Lead II, then the QRS mean vector is either −30° or +150°. Between these two, the lead with the most positive deflection is closest to the QRS mean vector. Therefore, if Lead III has the largest positive deflection, Lead III is closest to the QRS mean vector. It is important to first determine which lead is most isoelectric before looking for the lead with the largest magnitude. If all leads are equal in their deflection, the QRS mean vector has an "indeterminate axis" [3].

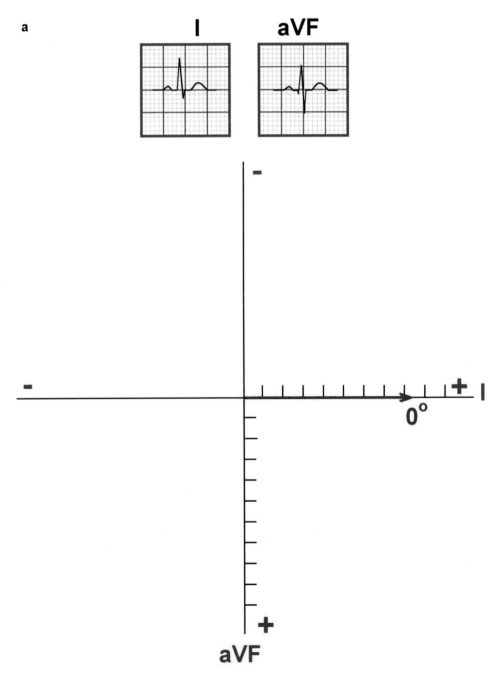

Fig. 3.4 (a) The QRS in aVF is a net zero since the positive and negative deflections are equal. Since the QRS in Lead I is a net positive, the QRS axis is aligned with Lead I, at 0°. (b) The QRS in aVF is a net zero (equal positive and negative deflections). Since the QRS in Lead I is a net negative, the QRS axis is aligned with Lead I, at 180°

Fig. 3.4 (continued)

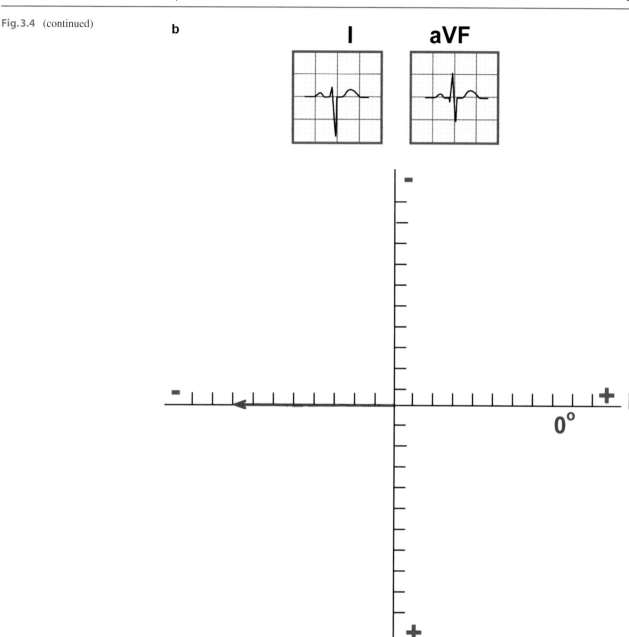

Graph Method QRS Determination

This method is relatively simple and fairly accurate; furthermore, it can be done mentally without the use of paper and pen. This method, like many others, uses the two perpendicular leads: I and aVF. Draw these two perpendicular leads on a graph paper, or alternatively mark on each lead equidistant lines to represent a ruler-like markings (Figs. 3.5, 3.6, 3.7, and 3.8). Examine Leads I and aVF on a 12-lead ECG to determine the net positive or negative deflection of the QRS complexes in each lead. Net deflection is the larger of the two deflections (R or S) minus the smaller deflection. Therefore, if the positive (upward) deflection in Lead aVF is 12 mm (each small square is 1 mm or 1 mV) and the net deflection is two,

then the net deflection is 10 positive units. Also, if the positive deflection in Lead I is seven while the negative deflection is four, the net positive deflection is three positive units.

By drawing perpendicular lines (red dashed lines in figure) from each line at the point of net positive deflection, the two lines will intersect. The QRS vector will be the line traversing the point of intersection of I and aVF to the point of the two drawn (red dashed) lines intersecting. An exact measurement will require a protractor; however, it is easy to estimate with a mere glance. After using this method, one gets accustomed to mentally envisioning the process without any actual plotting. For instance, if the net deflections in Leads I and aVF are positive, the mean

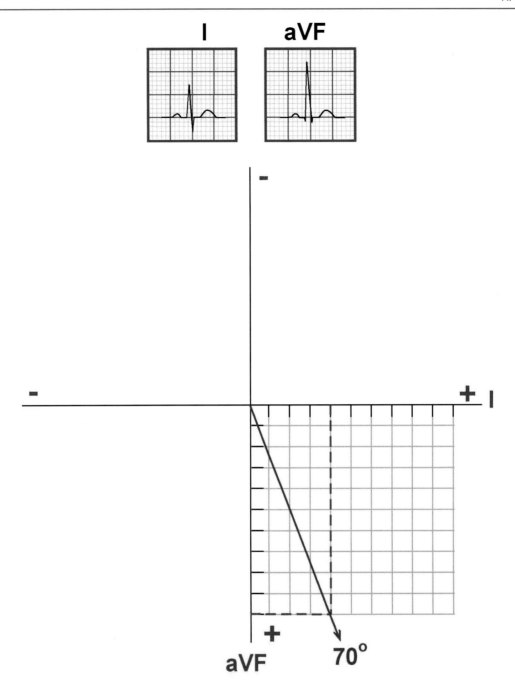

Fig. 3.5 QRS in Lead I is positive 7 and negative 3 mm; therefore the net QRS value in lead is positive 4. QRS in Lead aVF is positive 12 and negative 2 mm; therefore the net QRS value in lead is positive 10. By marking 4 on the positive end of Lead I and 10 on the positive end of Lead aVF, the perpendicular lines (red dashed line) intersecting produce a QRS axis (blue arrow) of 70°

QRS vector will be closer to 90° if the aVF QRS net positive deflection is much higher than that of I, and vice versa.

Formula-Based QRS Axis Determination

The mean vector can also be calculated based on the net voltage of the QRS complexes in Lead I and Lead III, using the

equation $\tan\theta = \dfrac{I + 2III}{\sqrt{3}I}$

θ is the angle subtended with the axis of Lead I. If the net voltage in Lead I is negative, the angle should be subtracted from 180° to find the QRS mean vector [3].

Axis Deviation

Normal axis varies by age (Appendix, Table 1). In a newborn, the QRS axis ranges from 60 to 180°, whereas it is −15° to 110° in adults [4, 5].

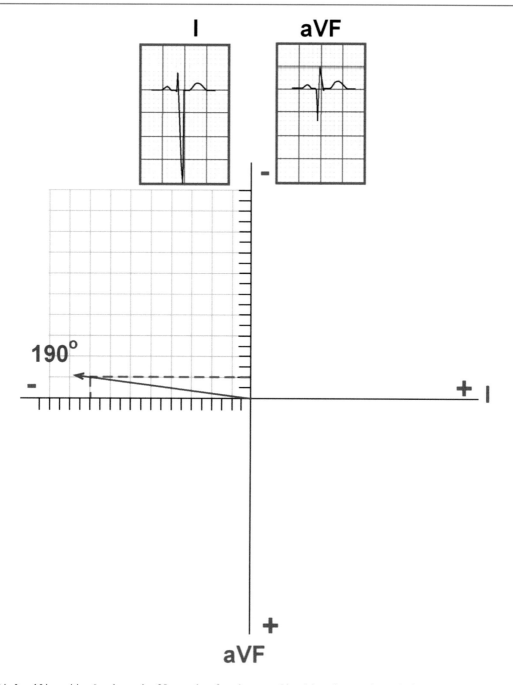

Fig. 3.6 QRS in Lead I is positive 6 and negative 20 mm; therefore the net QRS value in lead is negative 14. QRS in Lead aVF is positive 5 and negative 7 mm; therefore the net QRS value in lead is negative 2. By marking 14 on the negative end of Lead I and 2 on the negative end of Lead aVF, the perpendicular lines (red dashed line) intersecting produce a QRS axis (blue arrow) of 190°

QRS axis outside these ranges is abnormal (axis deviation), which could be right or left axis deviation.

Right Axis Deviation

A right axis deviation occurs when the QRS axis is greater than the upper limit of QRS axis range for age (110–180°) (Fig. 3.6). After 3 months and beyond, a right axis deviation is considered when the axis is more than 115° and usually no more than 180°.

Differential diagnosis of right axis deviation includes: right ventricular hypertrophy, right bundle branch block

secondary to surgery, hyperkalemia or drug toxicity such as sodium channel blockers, dextrocardia, WPW, and congenitally corrected transposition of the great vessels.

Left Axis Deviation

Left axis deviation is diagnosed when the QRS axis is −15 to 270° in adults and 0–270 in children (Fig. 3.7).

Differential diagnosis of left axis deviation includes left ventricular hypertrophy, left bundle branch block [2], lateral wall infarction as seen in children with anomalous left coronary artery from pulmonary artery, paced ventricular rhythm,

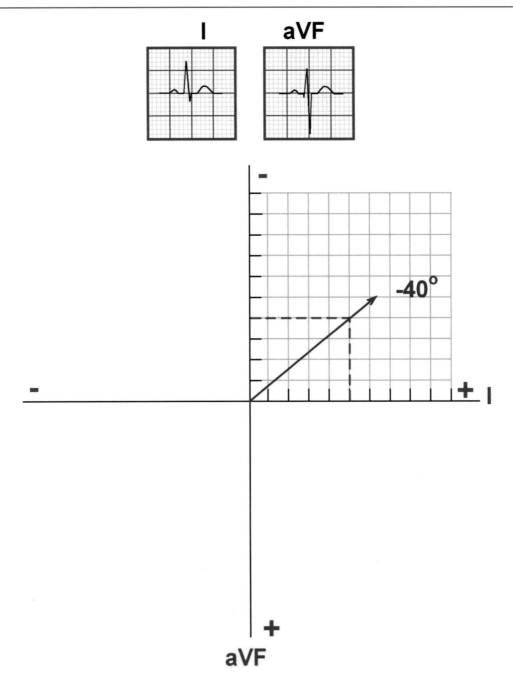

Fig. 3.7 QRS in Lead I is positive 7 and negative 2 mm; therefore the net QRS value in lead is positive 5. QRS in Lead aVF is positive 5 and negative 10 mm; therefore the net QRS value in lead is negative 5. By marking 5 on the positive end of Lead I and 4 on the negative end of Lead aVF, the perpendicular lines (red dashed line) intersecting produce a QRS axis (blue arrow) of −40°

ventricular inversion, and pectus excavatum due to clockwise rotation of the heart rendering the left ventricle more posterior and superior.

Superior Axis Deviation

Superior axis (negative deflection in Leads I and aVF) (Fig. 3.8) is seen in children with atrioventricular septal defect due to inferior displacement of the conduction pathways by the atrial ventricular septal defects. Patients with tricuspid atresia also have superior axis deviation due to hypoplastic right ventricle leading to diminutive or even absent right-sided forces. The ECG will show a left and superior axis deviation in nearly 90 % of tricuspid atresia with normally related great arteries. Fifty percent of patients with tricuspid atresia and d-TGA will also have QRS axis between 0 and −90°.

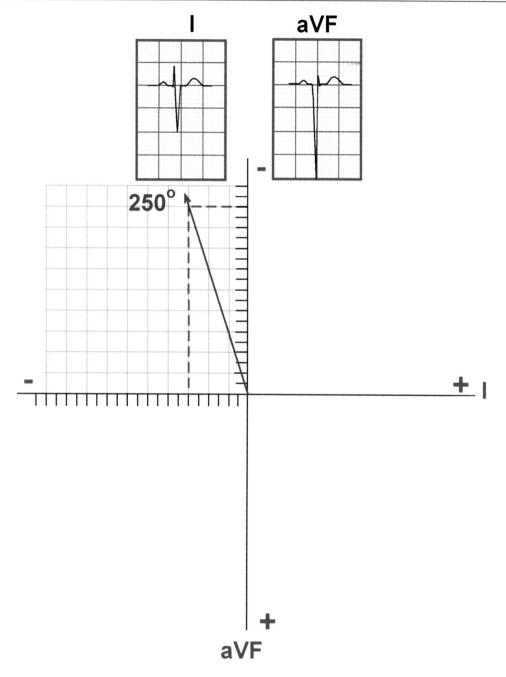

Fig. 3.8 QRS in Lead I is positive 4 and negative 10 mm; therefore the net QRS value in lead is negative 6. QRS in Lead aVF is positive 2 and negative 20 mm; therefore the net QRS value in lead is negative 18. By marking 6 on the negative end of Lead I and 18 on the negative end of Lead aVF, the perpendicular lines (red dashed line) intersecting produce a QRS axis (blue arrow) of 250°

T-Wave Mean Vector

In the frontal plane the T-wave mean vector can be calculated similarly to the QRS mean vector and is usually oriented in the same direction. The deviation between the QRS complex and the T wave can be an important metric, called the QRS-T angle. In infancy, this angle is extremely variable, but its upper limit is approximately 60° past the age of 6 months [4, 6].

The T wave should be positive in Leads I and II after day 2. It should be positive in Lead aVF after 5 days and should be negative in Lead aV_R at all ages [2].

Axis Abnormalities in Dextrocardia

Dextrocardia refers to the rightward orientation of the cardiac apex with reversal of anatomic ventricular left-right relationship, also referred to as mirror-image dextrocardia [7]. The right ventricle remains anterior but is to the left of the left ventricle. This is in contrast to dextroposition or dextroversion, where the ventricles remain in a normal right-left relationship to each other with the entire ventricular mass shifted into the right chest. Furthermore, with dextroposition there is also a degree of counterclockwise rotation (as viewed from apex) which results in the left ventricle being anterior to the right ventricle [7]. Since the degree of dextroposition can vary, the ECG findings are somewhat variable and are not as typical as with mirror-image dextrocardia.

Dextroposition

The major ECG effect of dextroposition is on the precordial leads: anterior V_2–V_4 have small Q waves and tall R waves (similar to V_6 in normal hearts) and the QRS amplitude progressively decreases from V_1 to V_6 (Fig. 3.9). The P-wave axis remains normal and Q waves are present in Leads I, V_5, and V_6 (same as levocardia). Ventricular hypertrophy can be difficult to assess due to the variable degree of ventricular rotation.

Dextrocardia

When an ECG is performed per standard technique with the chest leads arranged on the left chest, several findings will indicate mirror-image dextrocardia (Fig. 3.10). The P axis will be +90 to +180°, indicating a sinus node oriented on the left side of the heart. [2] No Q waves will be seen in Leads I and V_6. When right chest leads are recorded, the total voltage in Lead V_3R or V_4R is larger than the total voltage in Lead V_3 or V_4. Furthermore, if all right chest leads are recorded (V_1, V_3R through V_7R), the QRS morphologies in these leads should look the same as those found recording the left chest leads in a normally positioned heart. Q waves will be present in V_5R and V_6R.

Important points to remember when assessing ventricular position by ECG:

1. Gross ventricular orientation is best determined from the precordial leads.
2. Normal levocardia characteristically shows low or negative voltages in right chest leads (V_4R–V_2) with positive voltages of higher amplitude in mid and left chest leads.
3. The left ventricle is usually located on the same side as the precordial leads that show Q waves. Q waves represent septal depolarization which occurs from the morphologic LV to the RV.

Axis Abnormalities in Heterotaxy

Heterotaxy is a congenital disorder which encompasses a broad spectrum of complex cardiac lesions including a variety of congenital heart abnormalities in addition to abnormal visceral arrangement [8, 9]. Heterotaxy may include either right or left atrial isomerism (right or left bilateral sidedness of atria). This may result in an abnormal location of the sinus node, thus changing the location of the cardiac pacemaker and demonstrating on ECG by an abnormal P-wave axis.

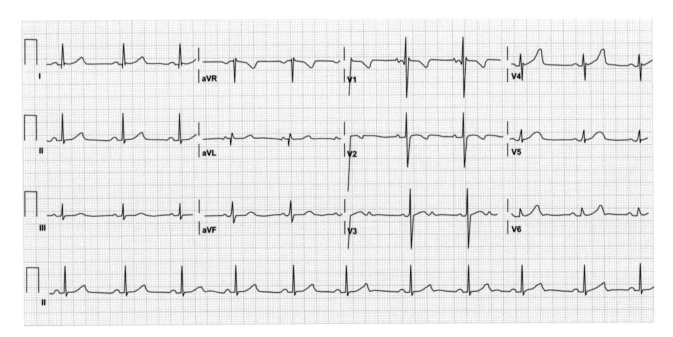

Fig. 3.9 Dextroposition, 12-lead ECG showing small Q wave and tall R wave with progressively decreasing amplitude of the R wave from right to left chest leads. Note that the P-wave axis is normal with Q waves in Leads I, V_5, and V_6

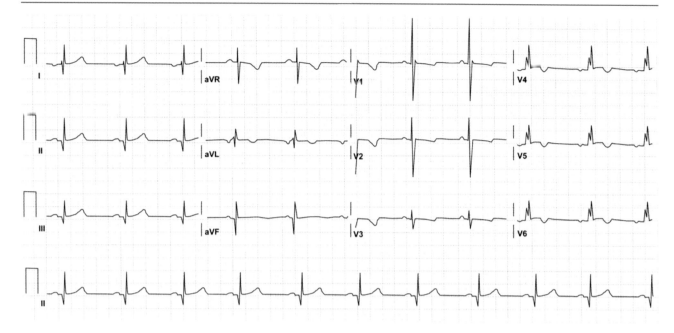

Fig. 3.10 Twelve-lead ECG from an infant with mirror-image dextrocardia. Note the absence of Q waves in Leads V_5 and V_6. There is a progressive decrease in amplitude from V_1 to V_6. Leads 1, V_5, and V_6 show an rSR pattern typical of this lesion

Electrocardiographic Findings

In right atrial isomerism, bilateral right atria are often present and there may be two sinus nodes. In such cases, competition between the sinus nodes may occur with two P waves (one positive while the other negative in Lead I), each having a slightly different rate [10]. Most children with right atrial isomerism have sinus rhythm and normal P-wave axis as the right-sided sinus node is usually the dominant atrial pacemaker [11] . Patients with dominant left-sided sinus node demonstrate a southwest P-wave axis (90–180°) on a 12-lead ECG [11, 12].

In left atrial isomerism, there may be absent sinus node and the P wave is noted to have an abnormal axis, usually a superior axis (−90) suggesting a low atrial pacemaker [10, 11]. In addition, patients can present with sinus node dysfunction, atrial fibrillation, and atrial flutter [13].

References

1. Kuhn L, Rose L. ECG interpretation part 1: understanding mean electrical axis. J Emerg Nurs. 2008;34:530–4. doi:10.1016/j.jen.2008.01.007.
2. Schwartz PJ, Garson A, Paul T, et al. Guidelines for the interpretation of the neonatal electrocardiogram: a task force of the European Society of Cardiology. Eur Heart J. 2002;23:1329–44. doi:10.1053/euhj.2002.3274.
3. Singh PN, Athar MS. Simplified [correction of simlified] calculation of mean QRS vector (mean electrical axis of heart) of electrocardiogram. Indian J Physiol Pharmacol. 2003;47(2):212–6.
4. Davignon A, Rautaharju P, Boisselle E, et al. Normal ECG standards for infants and children. Pediatr Cardiol. 1980;1:123–31. doi:10.1007/BF02083144.
5. Tipple M. Interpretation of electrocardiograms in infants and children. Images Paediatr Cardiol. 1999;1:3–13.
6. Rautaharju PM, Davignon A, Soumis F, et al. Evolution of QRS-T relationship from birth to adolescence in Frank-lead orthogonal electrocardiograms of 1492 normal children. Circulation. 1979;60:196–204. doi:10.1161/01.CIR.60.1.196.
7. Garson A. The electrocardiogram in infants and children: a systematic approach. Philadelphia: Lea & Febiger; 1983.
8. Park MK, Chamber Localization. How to read pediatric ECGs. 4th ed. Philadelphia: Mosby, Inc; 2006. p. 146–55.
9. Blieden LC, Moller JH. Analysis of the P wave in congenital cardiac malformations associated with splenic anomalies. Am Heart J. 1973;85:439–44.
10. Momma K, Linde LM. Abnormal P wave axis in congenital heart disease associated with asplenia and polysplenia. J Electrocardiol. 1969;2:395–405.
11. Wren C, Macartney FJ, Deanfield JE. Deanfield, cardiac rhythm in atrial isomerism. Am J Cardiol. 1987;59:1156–8.
12. Kim S-J. Heterotaxy syndrome. Korean Circ J. 2011;41:227–32.
13. Levine JC, Walsh EP, Saul JP. Radiofrequency ablation of accessory pathways associated with congenital heart disease including heterotaxy syndrome. Am J Cardiol. 1993;72:689.

Cardiac Conduction System

Christopher Bugnitz and Jessica Bowman

In order to understand the pediatric electrocardiogram, one must first understand the normal path of electrical conduction in the heart. In the structurally normal heart, the cardiac impulse is automatically generated by the pacemaker of the heart, the sinus node, and terminates in the ventricular myocardium. This chapter will discuss the anatomy and physiology of everything in between.

Sinus Node

The cardiac impulse begins in the sinus node, which historically, was the last component of the conduction system to be discovered. Discoveries actually began in 1839 with Jan Evangelista Purkinje, who found his famous fibers but believed that they were nonconducting cartilaginous structures. By the 1880s, Walter Gaskell knew that the cardiac impulse was generated at the sinus venosus but did not identify the specific source. Wilhelm His discovered his bundle in 1893. Sunao Tawara found the "complex knoten" known as the atrioventricular node in 1906. Finally, Arthur Keith and Martin Flack, an anatomist and medical student, respectively, identified the sinus node in 1907, thus completing the cardiac conduction system. Thomas Lewis later proved, using primitive electrocardiography, that the sinus node was the pacemaker of the heart [1].

The sinus node is a 10–20 mm by 5 mm mass located at the lateral aspect of the superior vena cava-right atrial junction just beneath the epicardium. Embryologically, it begins as a horseshoe-shaped structure in fetal life but morphs into

a crescent structure by birth. In 90 % of people, it is located just inferior to the crest of the right atrial appendage, whereas in 10 % it extends across the terminal crest. The so-called head of the sinus node courses toward the interatrial groove, while its tail extends toward the inferior vena cava [2].

There are three distinct sinus node cell types identified by histology: nodal cells, transitional cells, and atrial muscle cells. Nodal cells are small, ovoid, and pale when stained with hematoxylin and eosin. They are poorly striated and have fewer mitochondria than contractile myocytes, which makes sense from a functional standpoint, given that they are not responsible for contraction and therefore require less energy. Nodal cells are grouped together in a complex fibrous meshwork of interconnecting fascicles. Transitional cells, as the name implies, share properties of nodal and atrial myocytes. They bridge the gap between the nodal and atrial myocytes, allowing impulse propagation between the two [3].

Internodal and Interatrial Conduction

Internodal and interatrial depolarization travels from the sinus node to the left atrium and atrioventricular node (AV node) via internodal tracts. Heated debate has occurred over the years as to whether these tracts contain specialized myocytes [4]. The current evidence indicates that they are not histologically different but are the preferred route of conduction due to optimal muscle fiber orientation, thickness, and geometry. A study of cardiac specimens conducted by James in 1963 showed that the preferred pathways contained an abundance of Purkinje fibers, mixed with other cells including fat cells. In the end, there are three distinct pathways of conduction between the sinus and AV node and between the right and left atrium [3].

James described the course of the internodal tracts in great detail. The anterior internodal tract courses anteriorly from the sinus node along the superior vena cava and anterior wall of the right atrium to Bachmann's bundle, where it

C. Bugnitz, MD
Department of Cardiology, Nationwide Children's Hospital, 700 Children's Drive, Columbus, OH 43205, USA
e-mail: Christopher.burgnitz@nationwidechildrens.org

J. Bowman, MD (✉)
Department of Pediatrics, The Ohio State University/Nationwide Children's Hospital, 700 Children's Drive, Columbus, OH 43205, USA
e-mail: Jessica.bowman@nationwidechildrens.org

© Springer International Publishing Switzerland 2016
R. Abdulla et al. (eds.), *Pediatric Electrocardiography: An Algorithmic Approach to Interpretation*, DOI 10.1007/978-3-319-26258-1_4

divides into an anterior and posterior branch. The posterior branch conducts the cardiac impulse from the right to the left atrium. The anterior branch curves back toward the anterior portion of the interatrial septum, eventually terminating at the anterior superior margin of the AV node. The middle internodal tract, also known as Wenckebach's bundle, curves behind the superior vena cava, courses through the sinus intercavarum into the dorsal portion of the interatrial septum, and terminates in the superior margin of the AV node. The posterior internodal tract, or Thorel's bundle, courses posteriorly through the entirety of the crista terminalis and continues to the AV node via the Eustachian ridge [5].

Atrioventricular Junction

The atrial components of the atrioventricular axis are confined within three anatomic landmarks in the right atrial wall, which include the continuation of the Eustachian valve into the atrial myocardium, the tendon of Todaro (absent in two-thirds of people), and the hinge of the septal leaflet of the tricuspid valve. Collectively these boundaries are referred to as the triangle of Koch.

The AV node causes a delay in the cardiac impulse before it is propagated to the ventricular pathways. There are three distinct components of the AV junctional area: the atrial myocardium, the transitional cell zone, and the compact AV node. The transitional cell zone is a connection between the working atrial myocardium and the outer layer of the compact AV node. The compact AV node is located at the apex of the triangle of Koch, just beneath the right atrial posterior epicardium. At the base of the triangle is the coronary sinus. Below that is the cavo-tricuspid isthmus, a component of the most common form of atrial flutter. Between the coronary sinus and the hinge of the tricuspid valve is the septal isthmus, which contains the slow pathway into the AV node. The AV node lies directly next to the central fibrous body of the heart, which is formed by the fusion of the membranous septum with the rightward end of the area of fibrous continuity between the leaflets of the aortic and mitral valves in the roof of the left ventricle [4]. The distal continuation of the compact AV node is the penetrating portion of the AV bundle, or the bundle of His. In this region, the irregularly arranged fibers of the AV node become more organized and parallel, thereby forming the His bundle. This bundle subsequently dives into the ventricle through the fibrous central body, where it surfaces and then branches at the interface between the membranous and muscular ventricular septum in the left ventricular outflow tract [4, 6].

In the normal heart, the atrioventricular axis is the only myocardial structure that crosses the insulated plane of the AV junction. In patients with Wolff-Parkinson-White syndrome, there are other muscular connections between the right atrium and right ventricle, known as bundles of Kent, that allow for the electrical impulse to bypass the normal conduction pathway and preexcite the right ventricle before the impulse has had a chance to transmit through the AV junction. There are other accessory pathways that can exist between the His bundle and the crest of the ventricular septum. These are called Mahaim fibers and can also cause preexcitation. These accessory pathways are discussed further in later chapters.

Ventricular Conduction System

The ventricular conduction system is made up of the bundle branches and the Purkinje fibers. Conduction through this system is rapid due to specialized connexin proteins with high conductance properties [2].

Bundle Branches

The bundle of His divides into the right and left bundle branches at the crest of the muscular interventricular septum. The left bundle branch originates first from the common AV bundle and spreads like a web over the left ventricle, dividing into three branches, the anterior, middle, and posterior branches. The right bundle branch arises more distally from the common bundle and courses in the moderator band toward the right ventricular free wall. Its course from the common bundle along the right side of the ventricular septum begins subendocardially, then continues through the septal myocardium, and finishes subendocardially as it fans out into fascicles over the right ventricular myocardium [7]. From the fascicles in both ventricles, the impulse reaches the working myocytes via the Purkinje network.

Purkinje Fibers

First discovered by Jan Purkinje and described as nonconducting cartilaginous structures, these fibers are the final component of the cardiac conduction system. They are located in the subendocardium and extend transmurally. In human hearts, they are histologically not much different than adjacent ventricular myocytes. Interestingly, there are myocytes in the atrial myocardium and the pulmonary venous sleeves that resemble Purkinje cells and may be a nidus for ectopy [2].

Although their primary function is to conduct the cardiac impulse, Purkinje fibers can group together as false tendons and contribute, albeit minimally, to contraction.

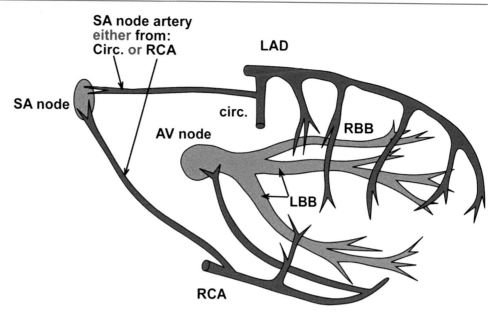

Fig. 4.1 Coronary blood supply to the cardiac conduction system. SA node is supplied either by a branch from the left circumflex artery or the right coronary artery, *not both as the illustration may imply*. AV node is supplied by the right coronary artery in most instances. *AV node* atrioventricular node, *Circ.* circumflex artery, *LBB* left bundle branch, *LCA* left coronary artery, *RBB* right bundle branch, *RCA* right coronary artery, *SA node* sinoatrial (sinus) node

Blood Supply

The sinus node receives its blood supply from the right coronary artery in 55–60 % of cases and the left circumflex coronary artery in 40–45 % of cases. The AV node is supplied by the AV nodal branch of the right coronary artery in about 80–85 % of people. In the other 10–15 %, it is supplied from the left circumflex artery. Due to its location in the superior muscular ventricular septum, the His bundle has a rich blood supply from the left anterior and posterior descending coronary arteries, making it well protected against ischemia [6] (Fig. 4.1).

Autonomic Control of Conduction

Autonomic input to the cardiac conduction system controls heart rate, also called chronotropy. An increase in heart rate is called positive chronotropy and a decrease is called negative chronotropy. It is important to understand that autonomic control of conduction is not merely the net sum of two opposing actions working independently at different parts of the conduction system, but rather it is an interactive process in which vagal and sympathetic nerves antagonize each other's ability to function. In terms of chronotropy, the autonomic nervous system exerts its main effects on the sinus and AV nodes. The sinus node is richly innervated with postganglionic adrenergic and cholinergic nerve terminals, containing more than a threefold greater density of beta-adrenergic and muscarinic cholinergic receptors than adjacent atrial tissue. Stimulation of beta-adrenergic receptors results in positive chronotropy. Stimulation of muscarinic receptors in the sinus node by acetylcholine produces the opposite effect, negative chronotropy. Acetylcholine also produces negative

chronotropy by prolonging intranodal conduction time. Similar effects are seen at the AV node [8].

It took many years to fully define the elusive cardiac conduction system. Each component plays a unique role in the transmission of the cardiac impulse. Knowing the anatomy and path of conduction will allow one to fully understand the components of the pediatric electrocardiogram.

References

1. Silverman ME, Hollman A. Discovery of the sinus node by Keith and Flack: on the centennial of their 1907 publication. Heart. 2007;93:1184–7. doi:10.1136/hrt.2006.105049.
2. Sizarov A, Moorman A, Pickoff A. Development and functional maturation of the cardiac conduction system. In: Moss and Adams' heart disease in infants, children, and adolescents: including the fetus and young adult. Philadelphia: Lippincott Williams & Wilkins; 2008. p. 348–71.
3. Waller BF, Gering LE, Branyas NA, Slack JD. Anatomy, histology, and pathology of the cardiac conduction system: part I. Clin Cardiol. 1993;16:249–52.
4. Anderson RH, Yanni J, Boyett MR, Chandler NJ, Dobrzynski H. The anatomy of the cardiac conduction system. Clin Anat. 2009;22:99–113. doi:10.1002/ca.20700.
5. James TN. The connecting pathways between the sinus node and a-V node and between the right and the left atrium in the human heart. Am Heart. 1963;J66:498–508. doi:10.1016/0002-8703(63) 90382-X.
6. Waller BF, Gering LE, Branyas NA, Slack JD. Anatomy, histology, and pathology of the cardiac conduction system: part II. Clin Cardiol. 1993;16:347–52.
7. Titus JL, Daugherty GW, Edwards JE. Anatomy of the normal human atrioventricular conduction system. Am J Anat. 1963;113: 407–15. doi:10.1002/aja.1001130305.
8. Liu Q, Chen D, Wang Y, Zhao X, Zheng Y. Cardiac autonomic nerve distribution and arrhythmia. Neural Regeneration Res. 2012;35:2834–41. doi:10.3969/j.issn.1673-5374.2012.35.012.

Cardiac Chamber Enlargement and Hypertrophy

5

Kaitlin L'Italien and Omar Khalid

Despite the development and widespread use of cardiac imaging modalities, such as echocardiography and magnetic resonance imaging, the ECG remains an important modality for the screening and assessment of cardiac chamber enlargement and hypertrophy. While there has been concern raised in recent years over lack of sufficiently diverse standardized or "normal" values, there is increasing awareness of expected variation between and within different populations. This chapter will attempt to summarize the key findings of cardiac enlargement or hypertrophy on ECGs while acknowledging limitations and areas of ongoing research.

To begin, historically the term "enlargement" was used to indicate either dilation of a chamber or hypertrophy of the heart muscle. The 1978 Bethesda Conference favored use of the term chamber enlargement, while the most recent recommendations from the AHA, ACCF, and HRS in 2009 predominantly refer to "ventricular hypertrophy" and "atrial abnormalities" [1]. We will use this terminology in discussing their characteristic ECG findings.

Atrial Abnormalities

Recognition that specific p wave abnormalities may indicate the presence of atrial anomalies has been well established. However, the terminology describing the abnormalities has changed through the years. In the beginning, the terms p-mitrale or p-pulmonale were used when it was noted that patients with mitral regurgitation or pulmonary hypertension each had characteristic p wave findings [1, 2]. These terms were replaced by left and right atrial enlargement to reflect the fact that other conditions can cause similar enlargement of the atria. Other terms describing p wave morphology have also been used. Descriptors such as atrial hypertrophy, atrial overload and interatrial conduction defects have been used to indicate that atrial dilation, hypertrophy, and abnormal conduction can all lead to p wave anomalies [1]. Thus, because there are multiple factors that can cause similar changes to p wave morphology, the less specific terms of right and left atrial abnormalities may be more accurate; on the other hand, right atrial enlargement continues to be the term more widely used.

Right atrial enlargement (RAE) commonly is associated with increased p wave amplitude and a rightward axis. Right atrial depolarization is responsible for the early part of the p wave, so when RAE is present, it typically manifests as a change in the height of the p wave, without any increase in p wave duration. If the p wave amplitude is greater than 2.5 mm in any lead, RAE is diagnosed (Fig. 5.1) [1–5]. These tall, narrow p waves are best seen in leads II, III, aVF, and V1. In addition, there may be a negative deflection of the p wave in V1, owing to the inferior location of the right atrium compared to the location of this lead [2].

RAE is commonly seen in congenital heart lesions, such as atrial septal defects, pulmonary stenosis, tricuspid valve anomalies, and tetralogy of Fallot. It should also be noted that while p wave duration is typically normal in RAE, it may be prolonged in patients with surgically repaired congenital heart disease, especially patients with single ventricle physiology [1]. RAE is also commonly seen in both acute and chronic pulmonary disease and has been transiently seen following episodes of supraventricular tachycardia [3].

K. L'Italien, MD
Department of Pediatric Cardiology, The Ohio State University/ Nationwide Children's Hospital, Columbus, OH 43205, USA

O. Khalid, MD (✉)
Department of Cardiology, Nationwide Children's Hospital, 700 Children's Drive, Columbus, OH 43204, USA
e-mail: Omar.Khalid@nationwidechildrens.org

© Springer International Publishing Switzerland 2016
R. Abdulla et al. (eds.), *Pediatric Electrocardiography: An Algorithmic Approach to Interpretation*,
DOI 10.1007/978-3-319-26258-1_5

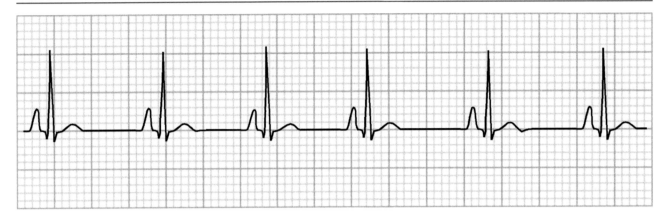

Fig. 5.1 Right atrial enlargement in limb lead II, note the peaked p wave with amplitude >2.5 mm

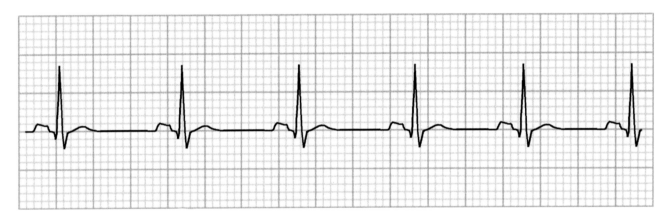

Fig. 5.2 Left atrial enlargement as seen in lead II, P waves are wide and notched with a duration >0.12 s

Left atrial enlargement (LAE) is commonly associated with an abnormally wide p wave, with a duration of 0.12 s or more (at least three small boxes, Fig. 5.2) [1, 2]. This is due to the fact that the left atrium depolarizes after the right atrium and thus is responsible for the terminal portion of the p wave [3]. The p waves may have a notched appearance (with "two humps") corresponding to the early depolarization of the right atrium and the delayed depolarization of the left atrium. This is usually best seen in the extremity leads [1, 2]. In addition, patients with LAE may have a characteristic biphasic p wave in lead V1. Typically there is a small positive deflection, followed by a large negative deflection at least 1 mm or more in depth and at least 0.04 seconds long. This negative deflection is due to the left atrium being posteriorly located, and its voltage directed away from V1 [2, 3].

LAE may occur in a number of clinically important situations, including disorders of the mitral or aortic valves or with the cardiomyopathies [2]. LAE is also more commonly associated with conduction delays than RAE and often represents a delay in the specialized interatrial conduction pathway (Bachmann's bundle) [1]. In addition, LAE may also be seen in patients with coronary artery disease due to atrial conduction delays [2].

Ventricular Hypertrophy

Unlike p wave anomalies, which can be due to a number of different atrial irregularities, variations in the QRS complex are predominantly caused by ventricular hypertrophy (i.e., *not* caused by dilation). Both the left and right ventricles depolarize at the same time. This stands in contrast to the depolarization of the atria, in which the right atrium depolarizes first, followed by the left. Unlike atrial abnormalities, which may be marked by a change in the duration of the p wave, ventricular hypertrophy does not typically affect the duration of the QRS complex [1, 2].

Ventricular hypertrophy is commonly signaled by changes in the amplitude of the QRS complex, compared to normal values and patterns. Therefore, knowledge of normal QRS morphology is essential for understanding how it is expected to change in conditions of ventricular hypertrophy. Because the left ventricle has a greater mass than the right ventricle, it is electrically dominant at baseline. Thus, leads placed on the right side of the chest will typically manifest a QRS complex with a prominent S wave, indicating that the larger mass is depolarizing on the left side. Conversely, leads placed on the left side of the chest will often have a prominent R wave, due to the larger forces generated by the left ventricle [2]. In addition to changes in QRS complex, changes in T wave morphology and axis deviation are also seen with ventricular hypertrophy [1–3, 6]. The specific changes seen with right ventricular and left ventricular hypertrophy are detailed below.

Right Ventricular Hypertrophy (RVH)

Right ventricular hypertrophy (RVH) is an increase in mass or thickness of the right ventricle. This causes an increase in right ventricular electrical forces relative to the normal heart, which causes a shift in the prominent positive forces to the right side [1–3]. Over the years, a number of specific criteria have been suggested to help characterize the ECG findings associated with RVH. While the majority of these criteria were proposed in the first half of the twentieth century and were based primarily on autopsy data, they remain valid. In some cases, echocardiogram has also been used to confirm the data; however, it is less helpful in confirming RVH than in left ventricular hypertrophy due to the complex three-dimensional shape of the right ventricle and the challenge of obtaining a measurement of the right ventricular free wall thickness [1]. The following are criteria that are used in the electrocardiographic diagnosis of RVH in children, and as such are based upon normative values for age:

1. *R wave amplitude in V1 >98 % for age:* If the amplitude of the R wave in lead V1 is greater than the 98 % for age, this may indicate RVH [3, 6]. A "normal" QRS complex in V1 typically has a smaller R wave and a more prominent S wave (Fig. 5.3). Again this is due to the fact that in a normal heart, the left ventricle has a larger mass and provides a larger, negative, force in the right chest leads. In RVH, the right ventricular mass is greater than expected, leading to a more positive vector (Fig. 5.4). Thus, the R wave will be greater than expected in the right chest leads [2, 3].

   It also should be noted that in RVH, the R waves are usually 0.04 s or longer in duration. If there is an R wave in V1>98 %, but it is shorter than 0.03 s, this may not be due to RVH but rather caused by focal septal hypertrophy. A brief, tall R wave can also be seen in muscular dystrophy [3].

   In general, the finding of an R wave amplitude >98 % for age in V1 is considered a fairly specific but nonsensitive measure. This is due to the relative dominance of the left ventricular mass compared to the right, and that there may be cases of right ventricular hypertrophy that still do not shift the balance of forces enough to cause a tall R wave [1].

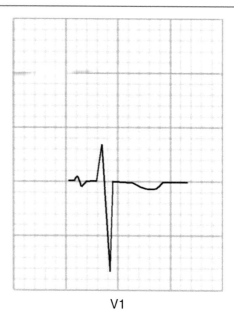

Fig. 5.3 Right chest lead (*V1*) in a normal child. The R wave is small with a more dominant S wave due to the smaller right ventricular mass when compared to the left ventricular mass

2. *S wave amplitude in V5, V6 >98 % for age:* If the depth of the S wave in V5 or V6 is greater than the 98 % for age, this may indicate RVH (Fig. 5.4) [3]. This criterion makes intuitive sense as it is essentially the inverse of the first criterion; if increased right ventricular mass causes an increase in the amplitude of R wave in the right-sided chest leads, it should also cause an increase in the amplitude of the S wave in the left-sided chest leads. This is considered a sensitive, but less specific, sign of RVH. Conditions other than RVH that can result in large S waves in the left-sided chest leads include focal left ventricular hypertrophy of the septum and left anterior hemiblock [3].

3. *R to S ratio in V1:* If the ratio of R to S in V1 is greater than one, it is suggestive of RVH (Fig. 5.5, above) [2–4]. This criterion may be thought of as another variant on the theme of larger than normal right-sided forces increasing the positive deflection in the right-sided chest leads. Unlike the prior two criteria which relate the R and S waves to normative values, this criterion more directly relates the electrical forces of the right ventricle relative to left ventricle of a given patient. In the normal heart, there is a small R wave and a prominent S wave in V1, owing to the relative dominance of the left ventricle. This particular criterion demonstrates that RVH causes an increase in the R wave relative to the S wave.

4. *QR pattern in V1, V3R, or V4R:* A Q wave in V1, V3R, or V4R may be seen in RVH. In RVH, the hypertrophied right side of the septum causes a large posterior vector, which results in the Q wave in V1 (Fig. 5.5) [3]. In

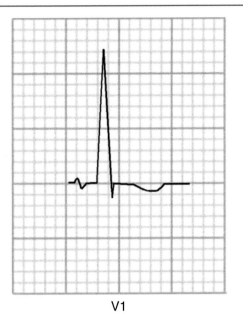
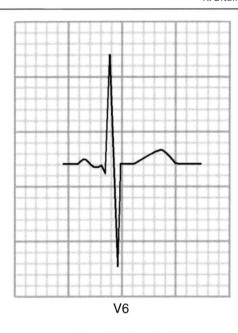

V1

V6

Fig. 5.4 An 8-year-old child with RVH. Note the tall R in *V1* and deep S wave in lead *V6*. The R/S ratio in lead V1 is greater than 1 supporting the diagnosis of RVH

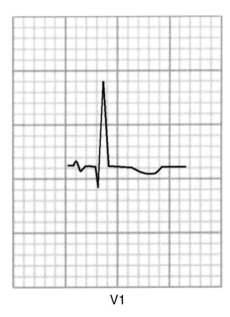

V1

Fig. 5.5 Deep Q waves in *V1*, suggestive of RVH

infants, the Q waves associated with RVH may only be 0.5–1 mm deep but may become more prominent in older children. However, as with most of these ECG criteria, the QR pattern is not only seen in RVH; it can be seen in ventricular inversion and in anterior myocardial infarctions, so it is helpful to use additional criteria to ensure the QR pattern is due to RVH. Of note, the QR pattern in RVH typically has a tall R wave, while the QR pattern seen in ventricular inversion or myocardial

infarction, the Q wave may be deeper and the R wave not as tall [3].

5. *ST depression and T wave inversions in the right precordial leads*: ST segment abnormalities and T wave inversions in the right sided leads are commonly seen with RVH [2, 3, 9]. As you recall, the "normal" T waves in the right precordial leads are upright at birth, but by 1 week of age, they become inverted. The T waves will remain inverted until prepuberty [6]. Given that the T waves are typically inverted during this time period, the finding of an upright T wave in a patient of this age is abnormal and may be a sign of RVH. Furthermore, the presence of an asymmetrically inverted T wave is also abnormal. The asymmetric T wave may have a slightly softer slope to its downward deflection and then a more severe, concave deflection of the terminal portion (Fig. 5.6). While this pattern was historically referred to as "strain" pattern, it is now recommended to be called "secondary ST-T abnormality" [1].

As with many of the other criteria, secondary ST-T wave abnormalities are not unique to RVH. T wave inversions have been transiently noted in patients during times of increased right ventricular pressure caused by upper airway obstruction and hypoxia. Of note secondary ST-T abnormalities in this situation will return to normal following alleviation of the source of increased RV pressure [1, 2]. In addition, abnormally upright T waves may be seen in situations causing left ventricular strain pattern in the left precordial leads (V5, V6); the inversion of the T waves in the left precordial leads may lead to a reciprocal flip of the T waves in the right precordial leads from inverted to upright [3].

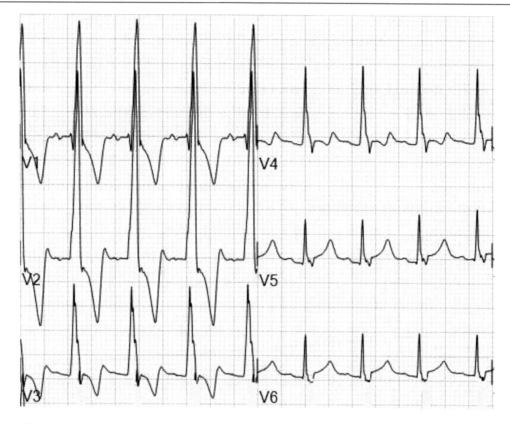

Fig. 5.6 Patient with prominent R waves in the right precordial leads and significant "secondary ST-T abnormality" as shown by the asymmetrically inverted T waves. These changes were formerly referred to as "strain" pattern

6. *RsR' pattern in V1 with a normal QRS duration (<0.12 s)*: RsR' pattern is commonly seen in mild RVH [1–3]. The RsR' pattern in V1 is sensitive, but not specific; it may be seen in normal children and those with incomplete RBBB. However, in the case of RVH, the R' portion is generally more prominent. Specifically, an R' of >15 mm in a child under 1 year of age or >10 mm in a child over 1 year of age, is suggestive of RVH (Fig. 5.7) [3]. The RsR' is thought to suggest volume overload and is commonly seen in patients with hemodynamically significant atrial septal defects (ASD).

7. *Right axis deviation*: Persistent right axis deviation in patients over 3 months old is associated with RVH [1–3, 6, 12]. It is often used as "supporting evidence" for patients who have other finds associated with RVH. For example, in patients with an RsR' pattern in V1 or a deep S wave in V5 or V6, a right axis deviation may lead one closer to a diagnosis of RVH and away from alternate causes.

8. *Right atrial enlargement (RAE)*: This may be viewed as a supporting sign of RVH, as many conditions commonly leading to RVH also often cause right atrial anomalies (RAE) or overload. Conditions such as pulmonary stenosis, hemodynamically significant ASDs, tetralogy of Fallot, or pulmonary hypertension will often demonstrate

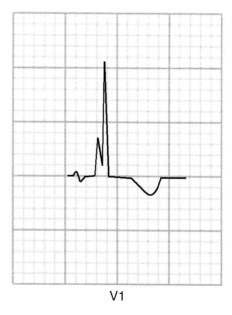

V1

Fig. 5.7 The rsR' pattern of RVH with a significant R'. QRS duration is normal which rules our right bundle branch block

RAE in addition to the aforementioned signs of RVH. An important exception to this rule is mitral stenosis—which often demonstrates ECG findings of associated RVH and left atrial anomalies [2].

Left Ventricular Hypertrophy (LVH)

Historically, the diagnostic criteria for *left ventricular hypertrophy* (LVH) were based upon measurements of QRS voltages. While the first studies were based upon R and S voltages in the limb leads I and III, in the late 1940s, Sokolow and Lyon proposed a now widely used criterion for determining LVH in the adult population by taking the sum of the S in V1 and the R wave in V5 or V6. Alternate criteria include the Cornell voltage, which is the sum of the S wave in V3 and the R wave in aVL, and the point score of Romhilt and Estes, which looks at abnormalities in the QRS axis and duration, QRS onset to peak time, P wave and ST segment morphology, as well as QRS amplitude. The sensitivity for these criteria is generally low, while the specificity is high. Also data has shown that patients who meet criteria for LVH by one set of criteria often do not meet it using another. In a large study of adult patients with hypertension, only 11 % of patients who met criteria for LVH by either the Sokolow and Lyon criteria or the Cornell criteria met it for both [1].

Another issue of predominately using voltage criteria is that QRS voltages are influenced by age, gender, race, body habitus, and athletic conditioning [1, 7–10]. In the adult population, QRS voltages tend to decrease with advancing age, and the commonly used voltage criteria apply to adults over 35 years old. Standards for 16–35 years old have not yet been established. Gender differences in QRS voltages are widely established. Adult women have lower upper limit of QRS voltage than men, and these gender differences appear to

arise during adolescence [1, 11]. People of African descent have higher normal QRS voltages than people of European descent, and people of Hispanic descent have lower voltages [6, 7]. Obese patients may have a decreased QRS voltage due to their larger amounts of adipose providing an insulating effect and causing an increased distance from the heart to the chest wall electrodes, which may underrepresent the QRS voltages [1, 13].

At time of publication, insufficient studies had been done to develop new "normative" curves for adult or pediatric populations—current "standards" do not yet account for the recently demonstrated differences in age, race, gender, and body habitus. Thus, the following guidelines are not absolute for all people and must be taken into account with a greater understanding of how age, race, gender, and body habitus may affect an individual compared to normative values. Nonetheless, the following criteria remain useful in the diagnosis of LVH in the pediatric population. As with the criteria described previously for right ventricular hypertrophy, the more criteria that are present, the stronger the case for LVH:

1. *R wave amplitude in lead V6 or S wave amplitude in lead V1 >98 % for age*: If either the height of the R wave in V6 or the depth of the S wave in V1 (or if the sum of the two) is greater than the 98th percentile for age, this should be described as "left ventricular hypertrophy by voltage criteria" (Figs. 5.8, and 5.9) [3]. Thinking again of the electrical force vectors generated by each ventricle, this makes intuitive sense—if there is an increased left

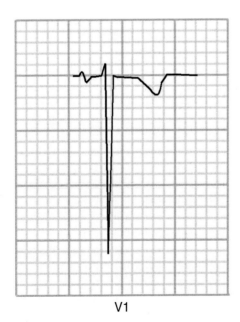

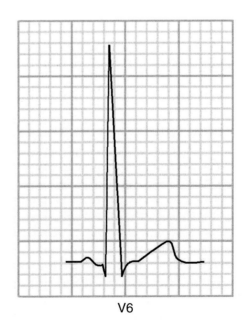

V1   V6

Fig. 5.8 An ECG from a 15-year-old male with voltage criteria suggestive of LVH, based upon R waves in V6 much greater than 98 % of normative values. The S in V1 is deep and supportive of a diagnosis of LVH

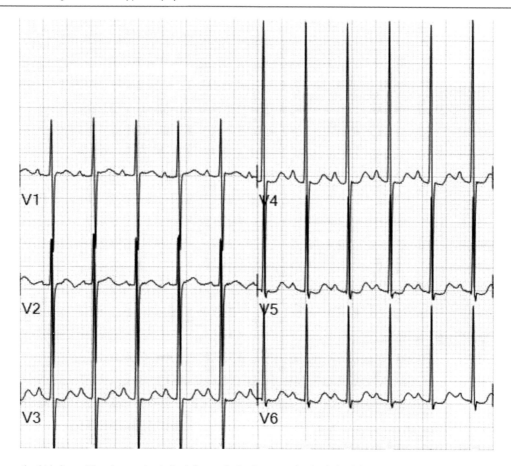

Fig. 5.9 A 1-month-old infant with voltage criteria for left ventricular hypertrophy, both the S in V1 and the R in V6 are above the 98 % for age

ventricular mass, this would lead to a stronger electrical force from the left ventricle and an exaggeration of the typical QRS pattern: taller R waves in the left lateral chest leads and deeper S waves in the right chest leads.

The terminology LVH by "voltage criteria" rather than simply "LVH" stems from the variables described in the introduction above. There are variations due to age, race, physical conditioning, body habitus, and gender that have been well described, and yet there are currently inadequate normative standards to sufficiently account for such variations. Thus, rather than jumping to a diagnosis of LVH on the basis of ECG findings alone, the terminology "voltage criteria for LVH" is less definitive and allows for alternate diagnostic modalities to confirm a possibility of LVH [1].

2. *ST segment and T wave anomalies*: There are two types of T wave changes that may suggest LVH, and they may seem at first to be opposites: either large positive T waves with increased amplitude or asymmetrically inverted T waves can signify LVH [1–3]. In mild LVH, the positive T waves are increased in amplitude. The sign of more severe LVH is inverted T waves. Basically, T waves should be upright in V5 and V6 by 48 h of life. When the T waves are inverted in patients over 48 h of age, espe-

cially with asymmetric inversion, this is a highly reliable sign of LVH [3, 6, 11]. Classically, there is a trio of changes thought to indicate strain on the left ventricle: J point depression, downsloping depression of ST segment, and asymmetrical inversion of the T wave. These changes were referred to as "strain pattern." Such terminology is now discouraged, and the term "secondary ST-T abnormalities" is preferred (Fig. 5.10) [1].

3. *Q wave abnormalities*: Q wave changes with LVH may deepen the Q wave or may lead to the absence of a Q wave. When the Q waves are unusually deep in the inferior and lateral leads (II, III, aVF, V5, V6), this may be a sign of LVH. Specifically, deep Q waves may signify left ventricular dilation or septal hypertrophy due to an increased right anterior and superior QRS force (Fig. 5.11). Alternately, when there is LVH due to concentric thickening of the muscle, the QRS vector is shifted in a left-posterior direction, which shifts the initial forces more to the left and can cause the Q wave to disappear [3].

4. *Left atrial enlargement (LAE), left axis deviation, and prolonged QT intervals*: Each of these anomalies are often associated with LVH, but should not be used as a stand-alone criteria, rather as supporting evidence [1–3].

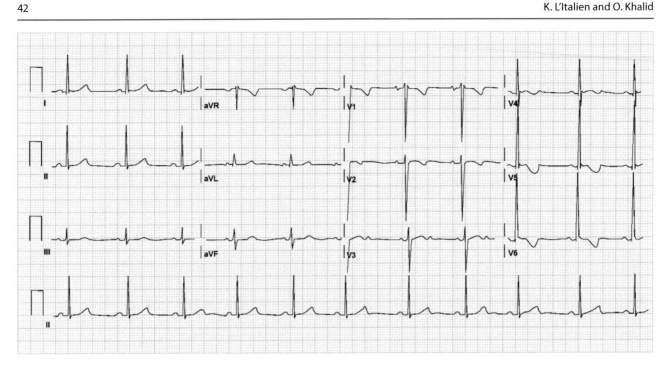

Fig. 5.10 ECG suggesting LVH by both voltage criteria in V6, and secondary ST-T abnormalities in the left chest leads

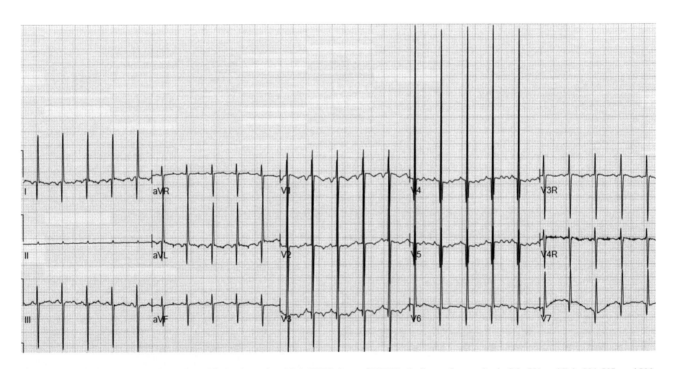

Fig. 5.11 ECG from a patient with tricuspid atresia, and multiple ECG signs of LVH including voltage criteria S in V1 and R in V4, V5, and V6. There are also prominent Q waves in the left-sided chest leads, as well as left axis deviation

Biventricular Hypertrophy (BVH)

1. *Abnormally large voltages in both left and right chest leads*: When criteria is met for either RVH or LVH and the reciprocal voltages in the left or right chest leads

exceed mean values, a diagnosis of BVH is made. For example, if a diagnosis of LVH is suspected and the R wave in V1 exceeds the mean for the patient's age, this meeds criteria for BVH. Often when one chamber is hypertrophic, the voltages from the other chamber will

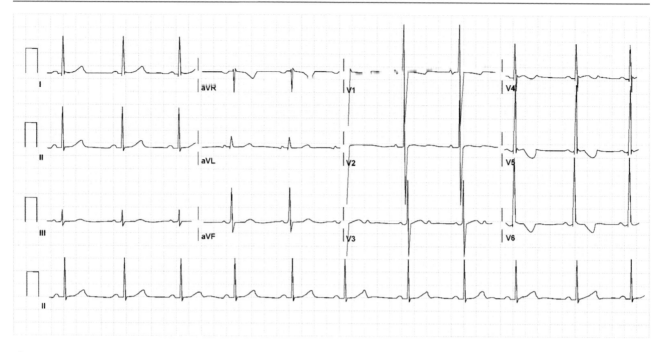

Fig. 5.12 In this ECG from a 1-week-old child pulmonary atresia, intact ventricular septum, there is electrocardiographic evidence of biventricular hypertrophy. Both the R and S waves in V1 are above-expected size, as well as the R in V6

seem small by comparison. When they do NOT seem small, this may be a sign of biventricular hypertrophy (Fig. 5.12).

2. *Sum of R + S >98 % in mid-precordial leads*: When the sum of the R and S waves in the mid-precordial leads exceeds the 98 % for age, this may be a sign of BVH. This is called the "Katz-Wachtel" criterion [3].

References

1. Hancock EW, et al. AHA/ACCF/HRS recommendations for the standardization and interpretation of the electrocardiogram. Part V: electrocardiogram changes associated with cardiac chamber hypertrophy. A scientific statement from the American Heart Association Electrocardiography and Arrhythmias Committee, Council on Clinical Cardiology; the American College of Cardiology Foundation; and the Heart Rhythm Society. JACC. 2009;53(11):992–1002.
2. Goldberger AL. Clinical electrocardiography: a simplified approach. 6th ed. Mosby: St. Louis; 1999.
3. Garson A. The electrocardiogram in infants and children: a systematic approach. Philadelphia: Lea & Febiger; 1983.
4. Davignon A, et al. Normal ECG standards for infants and children. Pediatric Cardiology. 1979/80;1:123–31.
5. Rijnbeek PR, et al. New normal limits for the paediatric electrocardiogram. Eur Heart J. 2001;22:702–11.
6. O'Connor M, et al. The pediatric electrocardiogram part 1: age-related interpretation. Am J Emerg Med. 2008;26:221–8.
7. Rautaharju P. Ethnic differences in ECG amplitudes in North American white, black, and hispanic men and women. J Electrocardiol. 1994;27:20–30.
8. Macfarlane PW, et al. Racial differences in the ECG-selected aspects. J Electrocardiol. 2014;47:809–14.
9. Uberoi A, et al. Interpretation of the electrocardiogram of young athletes. Circulation. 2011;124:746–57.
10. Di Paolo FM, et al. The athlete's heart in adolescent Africans. JACC. 2010;59(11):1029–36.
11. Dickenson D. The normal ECG in childhood and adolescence. Heart. 2005;91:1626–30.
12. Tipple M. Interpretation of electrocardiograms in infants and children. Images Paediatric Cardiology. 1999;1(1):3–13.
13. Da Costa W, et al. Correlation of electrocardiographic left ventricular hypertrophy criteria with left ventricular mass by echocardiogram in obese hypertensive patients. J Electrocardiol. 2008;41:724–9.

Heart Rate and Rhythm Disturbances

William Bonney

Introduction

Few sounds evoke a feeling of life and vitality more than the regular "thump-thump" of a human heartbeat. When a person is resuscitated from cardiac arrest and their pulse returns, the regular beeping of a bedside monitor is a calming sound that allows everyone in the room to breathe a sigh of relief. Conversely, abnormal heart rhythms may send a wave of anxiety through the bodies of medical providers, particularly those who lack a sense of familiarity with arrhythmias. With a little practice and by following a methodical step-by-step system, one can learn to recognize the various abnormal heart rhythms that are commonly encountered in pediatric patients.

The art of interpretation of a rhythm strip or a 12-lead ECG can be achieved through different methodologies; in this chapter, we present our favored method; in doing so, different methodologies are available for consideration [1–5].

Diagnostic Algorithm

The key to rapid and accurate arrhythmia recognition starts with identifying the "four R's."

- *R*ate
- *R*egularity
- *QR*S morphology
- *R*elationship of QRS and P waves

By simply knowing the first three, *r*ate, regularity, and *QR*S morphology, one can usually identify an arrhythmia

W. Bonney, MD
Department of Cardiology, Children's Hospital of Philadelphia,
34th Street and Civic Center Boulevard,
Philadelphia, PA 19104, USA
e-mail: BONNEYW@email.chop.edu

with 90 % accuracy before the 12-lead ECG is even completed. Careful interpretation of the last "R" will usually confirm the suspected diagnosis.

Step #1: Determine the Heart *R*ate

There are several methods for determining the heart rate. Each with their own pros and cons:

Big Box Method By using the 300:150:100:75:60 rule, a rough estimate of the heart rate can be obtained by counting the number of large boxes between two QRS consecutive complexes (measured R-R interval). The advantage of this method is that it is quick to apply and easy to memorize. The disadvantage is that it is not very accurate at faster heart rates.

Little Box Method A similar method using the little boxes gives a more accurate heart rate. This sequence is more accurate than the big box method, but also difficult to memorize. If a calculator is available, one can simply remember that each little box corresponds to 40 milliseconds and use the following formula:

$$\frac{60}{(\text{number of little boxes between } R - R) * (0.04)}$$

Alternatively and based upon the same principal, one can measure the HR by dividing 1,500 by the number of small boxes between two consecutive QRS complexes (RR interval) (Fig. 6.1a, b).

Tick Mark Method ECG paper is usually scored at the bottom with tick marks that denote three-second intervals. The heart rate can be estimated by counting the number of QRS complexes between two tick marks and multiplying by twenty. This method is fairly accurate for faster heart rates, but less accurate for slower heart rates.

© Springer International Publishing Switzerland 2016
R. Abdulla et al. (eds.), *Pediatric Electrocardiography: An Algorithmic Approach to Interpretation*,
DOI 10.1007/978-3-319-26258-1_6

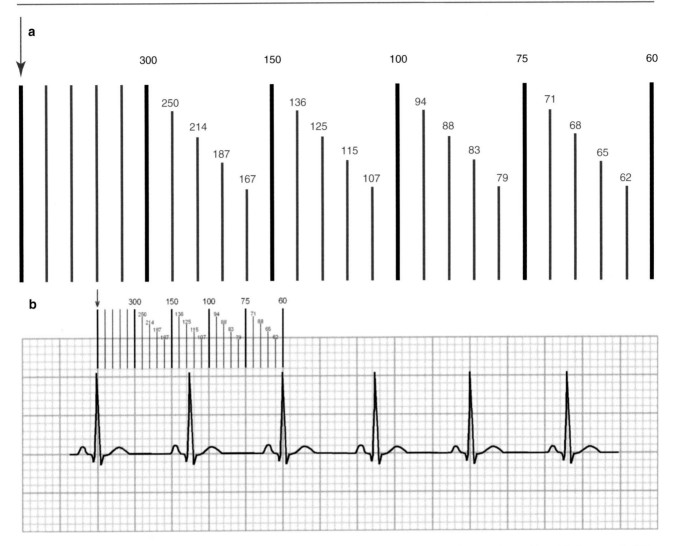

Fig. 6.1 (**a, b**) An illustration of a ruler used to measure heart rate. The *red arrow* is placed over the R in a QRS complex, typically in lead II. The heart rate is indicated by the ruler where the R of the subsequent QRS complex intersects with the ruler markings. The heart rate in (**b**) is 116–125 bpm

Whole ECG Method When run at standard 25 mm/s, a single-page ECG records ten seconds of the heart rhythm. The heart rate can be determined by counting the number of QRS complexes on the entire ECG and multiplying by six. Although this is the most time-consuming method, it is also the most accurate and can be applied without a calculator.

Step #2: Determine the *Regularity*

Heartbeats can be regular or irregular, and irregular heart rates can be further divided into *regularly irregular* (irregular but with a predictable pattern) vs. *irregularly irregular* (irregular but with no predictable pattern). Regularly irregular patterns are also sometimes referred to as "group beating." A common example is an AV Wenckebach pattern in which every fourth beat does not conduct. This effectively results in QRS complexes that occur in three-beat "groups" (Table 6.1).

Step #3: Determine the Q*R*S Morphology

QRS morphology is usually characterized as narrow or wide, with the former implying conduction through the AV node and His-Purkinje system and the latter implying that the rhythm travels outside these channels (i.e., ventricular origin or aberrant conduction). Of course, there are exceptions to both of these. It is important to obtain a full 12-lead ECG before declaring a rhythm to have wide or narrow QRS, as certain leads may be misleadingly narrow (example of ECG where V1 is narrow but other leads are clearly wide).

Comparison with a baseline ECG that is known to be in sinus rhythm can be extremely helpful. If a wide QRS in

Table 6.1

| Regular rhythms | Irregular rhythms | |
	Regularly irregular	Irregularly irregular
• Sinus rhythms • Atrial flutter (with a fixed AV conduction ratio) • Reentrant SVT • Atrial tachycardia • Junctional ectopic tachycardia • Ventricular tachycardia	• Sinus arrhythmia • Wenckebach (Mobitz I 2nd degree AV block) • PACs or PVCs in bigeminy/trigeminy • Junctional ectopic tachycardia (with sinus capture beats)	• Atrial fibrillation • Chaotic atrial tachycardia • Mobitz II 2nd degree AV block • Atrial flutter (with variable conduction)

tachycardia matches the wide QRS in sinus rhythm, then it is more likely to be a supraventricular tachycardia.

Lastly, wide vs. narrow QRS is more of a qualitative interpretation than a quantitative measurement. Infants, in particular, may have wide QRS rhythms with a QRS duration that is less than 80 ms.

Step #4: Determine the Relationship Between QRS and P Waves

The P waves are leading the QRS (typical of supraventricular and atrial arrhythmias)

The QRS complexes are leading the P waves (typical of ventricular arrhythmias and reentrant supraventricular tachycardia)

There is no discernable relationship (characteristic of ventricular or junctional arrhythmias).

Arrhythmia Classifications

Arrhythmias can be classified by the rate at which they occur (tachyarrhythmias vs. bradyarrhythmias), by their location (atrial, ventricular, or junctional), or by the underlying electrophysiologic mechanism that causes the arrhythmia. There are three basic arrhythmia mechanisms, namely, automaticity, reentry, and triggered automaticity.

Automaticity is most commonly observed within the sinus node, but similar behavior can occur outside the sinus node in the form of ectopic atrial or junctional rhythms. The classic features of automatic arrhythmias involve a direct correlation with sympathetic tone, a gradual "warm-up" and "cooldown" of rates, and an inability to terminate tachycardia with DC shock or pacing maneuvers.

Reentry, on the other hand, implies that electrical excitation traverses a circuitous "loop" within the cardiac tissue. This loop can consist entirely of atrial tissue (e.g., atrial flutter), both atrial and ventricular tissue (e.g., supraventricular tachycardia utilizing an accessory atrioventricular pathway), or purely ventricular tissue (e.g., ventricular tachycardia related to scars resulting from surgery to repair congenital heart disease). Reentrant rhythms tend to be very regular with a fixed heart rate. They start and stop abruptly and can be terminated with DC shock and/or pacing maneuvers.

Table 6.2 Arrhythmia classification

I. Sinus rhythm
   A. Normal sinus rhythm
   B. Sinus tachycardia
   C. Sinus bradycardia
   D. Sinus arrhythmia
II. Rhythms arising from the atrium
   A. Low atrial rhythm
   B. Wandering atrial pacemaker
   C. Atrial extrasystoles
   D. Supraventricular tachycardias
      1. Paroxysmal SVT (PSVT)
         (a) Paroxysmal SVT: WPW and tachycardia mediated by an accessory pathway (AVRT and ORT)
         (b) Paroxysmal SVT: atrioventricular nodal reentrant tachycardia (AVNRT)
      2. Ectopic atrial tachycardia (EAT)
      3. Multifocal atrial tachycardia and chaotic tachycardia
      4. Atrial fibrillation
      5. Atrial flutter
III. Rhythms arising from the ventricles
   A. Ventricular extrasystoles or premature ventricular contractions (PVCs)
   B. Ventricular escape rhythms ventricular tachycardia (VT)
   C. Ventricular fibrillation
IV. Rhythms arising from the AV junction
   A. Junctional ectopic tachycardia

Triggered automaticity shares features common to both reentrant and automatic arrhythmias. The torsades de pointes variety of ventricular tachycardia that is observed in long QT syndrome may have triggered automaticity as part of the underlying mechanism. The "triggers" are known as after depolarizations, and these may produce a premature extrasystole (PAC or PVC) that initiates tachycardia. Triggered automatic arrhythmias may be sensitive to catecholamines and also may show a warm-up and cooldown. However, they can also be terminated with DC cardioversion.

Alternatively, heart rhythms may be classified by the location in the heart from which they originate, namely, the atria, the ventricles, or the AV junction. There are examples of automatic, reentrant, or triggered arrhythmias originating from each of these three locations. For the remainder of this chapter, arrhythmias will be categorized according to location (Table 6.2).

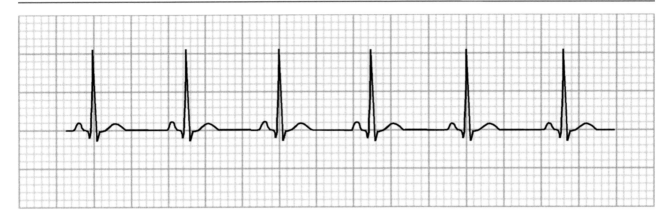

Fig. 6.2 Normal sinus rhythm, note that the P-QRS relationship is constant p wave preceding each QRS, normal p wave morphology, and a constant PR interval. The heart rate is within normal limits for a child

Sinus Rhythms

This includes sinus bradycardia, normal sinus rhythm, sinus tachycardia, and sinus rhythm with sinus arrhythmia. The defining characteristics of these rhythms include:

- a P wave precedes every QRS.
- a QRS complex follows every P.
- P wave morphology is normal (i.e., upright in lead I and AVL). Sinus P waves tend to have a rounded appearance.

Normal Sinus Rhythm

This is the classic example of an automatic rhythm. There is generally some variability to the rate, with subtle fluctuations that occur with respiration and postural changes. More pronounced changes may occur with exercise, stress, or virtually anything that elevates the endogenous catecholamine levels (Fig. 6.2 and Table 6.3).

There are three basic criteria for sinus rhythm:

1. A P wave must precede each QRS.
2. A QRS complex must follow each P wave.
3. The P wave morphology must be normal (i.e., positive in leads I and AVL).

Sinus Tachycardia

Sinus tachycardia (Fig. 6.3) is defined when the aforementioned three criteria for sinus rhythm are present, and the rate exceeds the normal value for a particular age (refer to table "Normal Heart Rates by Age"). There is no hard and fast upper limit for sinus tachycardia, and rates approaching 240 bpm are occasionally observed in premature infants in critical care situations. Pain, fever, infection, exercise, and

Table 6.3 Normal heart rate ranges by age

Age	HR (bpm)
1st week	90–160
1–3 weeks	100–180
1–2 months	120–180
3–5 months	105–185
6–11 months	110–170
1–2 years	90–165
3–4 years	70–140
5–7 years	65–140
8–11 years	60–130
12–15 years	65–130
>16 years	50–120

elevations in endogenous or exogenous catecholamine levels can all produce sinus tachycardia. Since AV conduction tends to become more brisk in these situations, the PR interval also shortens when the heart rate increases in sinus tachycardia. It is extremely rare for AV block to develop during sinus tachycardia when there is not already some existing AV block in the baseline state. Hence, a prolongation of the PR interval or the occurrence of 2nd-degree AV block during tachycardia would raise suspicion for an abnormal atrial tachycardia like ectopic atrial tachycardia or atrial flutter.

Sinus Bradycardia

Sinus bradycardia is defined when the three criteria for sinus rhythm are present and the heart rate is below the normal value for age (refer to table "Normal Heart Rates By Age"). True "sick sinus syndrome" is extremely rare in children and young adults with structurally normal hearts that have not been damaged by cardiac surgery. Sinus bradycardia usually results from excessive vagal tone or other endogenous and exogenous factors that slow the heart rate (Fig. 6.4).

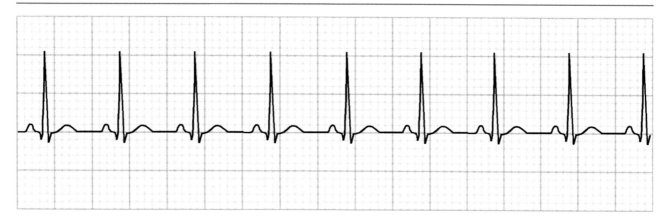

Fig. 6.3 Sinus tachycardia, note that the P-QRS relationship is constant p wave preceding each QRS, normal p wave morphology, and a constant PR interval. The heart rate is fast (150 bpm) for a child

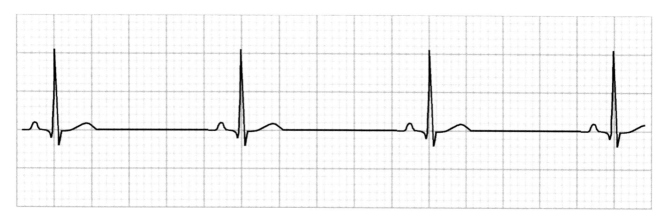

Fig. 6.4 Sinus bradycardia, note that the P-QRS relationship is constant p wave preceding each QRS, normal p wave morphology, and a constant PR interval. The heart rate is slow (60 bpm) for a child

---

The 4 R's of Sinus Rhythm

Rate: age dependent (may be as low as 40 in healthy teenagers or as much as 220 in neonates)

Regularity: regular

QRS: narrow

Relationship of QRS-P: P waves precede each QRS with normal P wave morphology and normal PR interval.

Sinus Arrhythmia

Sinus arrhythmia is the variation in the normal heart rate that occurs with respiration. Specifically, the heart rate increases with inspiration, and it decreases with expiration as the result of small fluctuations in vagal tone that occur as intrathoracic pressure varies. While this is a normal finding that occurs to some degree in every human, it is particularly pronounced in the young, especially in older toddlers and young school-aged children. When pronounced sinus arrhythmias occur, the heart rate may fluctuate with peaks in the low 100 s and nadirs in the 50s. On an ECG rhythm strip, the "peaks" of sinus arrhythmia may resemble short runs of atrial tachycardia. The trained ECG interpreter will identify sinus arrhythmia by a lack of change in the P wave morphology and also by the 3-s cycling that parallels respiration (Fig. 6.5).

Rhythms Arising from the Atrium

Low Atrial Rhythm

Low atrial rhythm is defined when the first two criteria for sinus rhythm are met, but point #3 is not because the P waves have an alternate morphology. Generally, the heart rate is below or near the low end of normal for the patient's age (50–70 bpm). These rhythms often originate from low in the right atrium near the mouth of the coronary sinus. This is considered to be a normal finding that is observed in up to 10 % of normal ECGs, particularly in people who have higher vagal tone and slower resting heart rates.

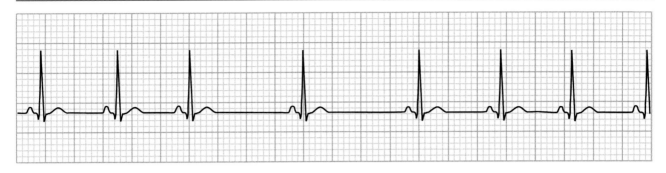

Fig. 6.5 Sinus arrhythmia, note that the P-QRS relationship is constant p wave preceding each QRS, normal p wave morphology, and a constant PR interval. The heart rate is variable in a cyclical fashion matching respiration. In this example, HR ranges from 75 to 100 bpm

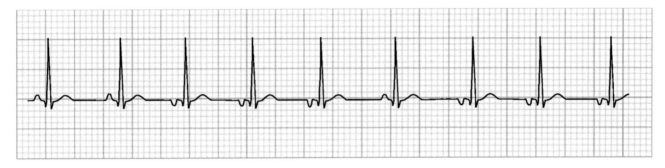

Fig. 6.6 Wandering atrial pacemaker, note how the P wave flips from upright to inverted for a few beats and then returns to normal as the heart rate accelerates during inspiration

Wandering Atrial Pacemaker

Wandering atrial pacemaker occurs when the rhythm alternates between two atrial sources. This occurs commonly during the nadir phase of a sinus arrhythmia. The P wave "flips" from upright to inverted for a few beats and then returns to normal as the heart rate accelerates during inspiration. In some cases, the rhythm during the nadir phase may be junctional rather than low atrial. All of these are essentially benign rhythms that do not result in any hemodynamic consequences or cause any symptoms (Fig. 6.6).

The 4 R's of Wandering Rhythms (Sinus Arrhythmia +/– Low Atrial Rhythm or Junctional Rhythm)
Rate: 40–80 bpm
Regularity: regularly irregular (bradycardia generally occurs every three seconds, coinciding with respiratory cycles)
QRS: narrow
Relationship of QRS-P: P waves precede each QRS with normal P wave morphology and normal PR interval. During periods of bradycardia, low atrial rhythm (inverted P waves) or junctional rhythm (no preceding P waves) may emerge.

When an atrial rhythm occurs at a rate that is in the upper-half of the normal range, this is called an "*accelerated atrial rhythm*," and if the rate is above the upper limit of normal, then the term "*atrial tachycardia*" applies. Unlike low atrial rhythms, these faster atrial arrhythmias are rarer and generally considered to be abnormal.

Atrial Extrasystoles

Atrial extrasystoles, also known as "premature atrial contractions" or PACs, are generally benign random occurrences. PACs occur in one of three forms:

- PACs with normal conduction (followed by a narrow QRS complex)
- PACs with aberrant conduction (followed by a wide QRS complex)
- Blocked PACs (no QRS complex follows the P wave)

When PACs occur, AV conduction varies according to the timing of these extrasystoles. PACs that occur late in the cardiac cycle generally conduct normally, while very early PACs that occur on top of the preceding T wave are more likely to show AV block. PACs are particularly common in newborns and infants. They may also be provoked by electrolyte imbalances, hyperthyroidism, or fever. In the hospital setting, PACs may be the result of mechanical "bumping" of atrial tissue that occurs when a venous catheter or other foreign body slips into the atrium (Fig. 6.7).

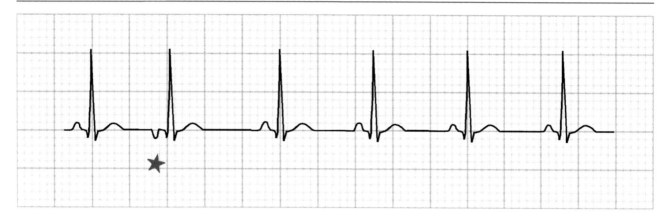

Fig. 6.7 Premature atrial contraction with normal AV conduction and QRS

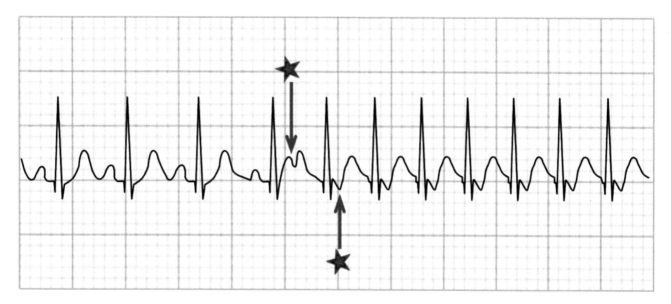

Fig. 6.8 Paroxysmal SVT, note the retrograde P waves after QRS complexes

Supraventricular Tachycardia

Rhythms originating from the upper chambers of the heart are referred to as supraventricular tachycardia (SVT), and these are by far the most common abnormal rapid heart rhythms encountered in children. Reentrant types like orthodromic reciprocating tachycardia (ORT) and AV nodal reentrant tachycardia (AVNRT) account for about 90 % of SVT seen in children and infants, while other types of SVT like atrial fibrillation, atrial flutter, and ectopic atrial tachycardia are rare in this population.

Paroxysmal SVT (PSVT)

In children, the most common types of SVT are reentrant. These are typically triggered by a critically timed PAC or PVC and generally continue for some time until terminated by block within the AV node, accessory pathway, or another critical part of the reentry loop. Hence, these types of SVT are episodic in nature, and they generally consist of longer runs. PSVT is the type of SVT that is most familiar to general practitioners, and the ability to terminate this arrhythmia with adenosine or vagal maneuvers is well known. PSVT is mediated by one of two mechanisms: dual pathways within the AV node (*AVNRT*) or an accessory pathway, distinct from the AV node, that serves as an electrical connection between the ventricle and atrium (*AVRT*). Clinically, these two types of SVT are indistinguishable. Both produce a regular, narrow QRS tachycardia. Both can be terminated by adenosine or vagal maneuvers. The same medications are generally used for maintenance antiarrhythmic therapy in both cases, and catheter ablation is an equally effective in permanently curing these two arrhythmias. There are, however, several ECG findings that help to distinguish the two (Figs. 6.8, 6.9, 6.10, and 6.11).

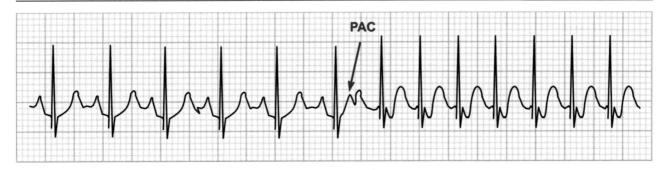

Fig. 6.9 SVT is initiated by a PAC (*upright* P wave). During tachycardia, retrograde P waves are visible in the early portion of the T wave, and they do not overlap with the QRS. This is typical of orthodromic reciprocating tachycardia using an accessory pathway

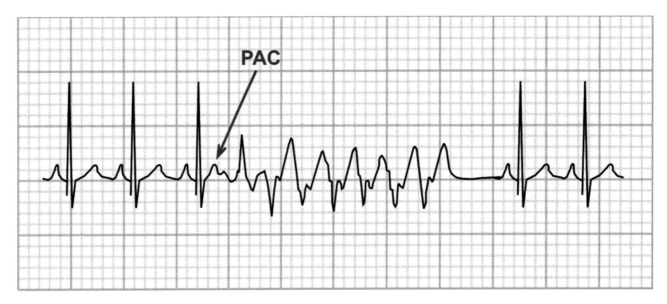

Fig. 6.10 SVT with aberrant conduction, this may appear very similar to VT. Note the PAC preceding the wide complex SVT due to aberrant conduction

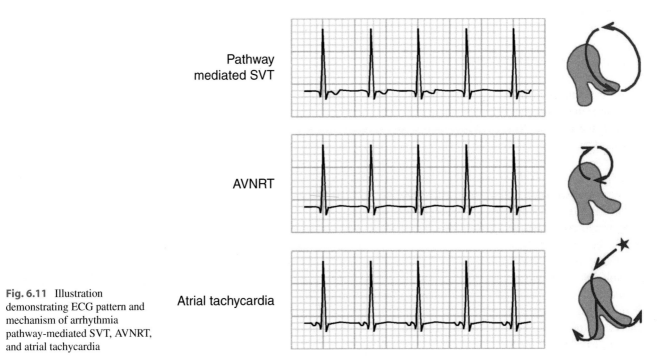

Fig. 6.11 Illustration demonstrating ECG pattern and mechanism of arrhythmia pathway-mediated SVT, AVNRT, and atrial tachycardia

The 4 R's of Paroxysmal SVT (AVNRT and Accessory Pathway-Mediated SVT)

Rate: usually 190–260 bpm

Regularity: regular

QRS: narrow

Relationship of QRS-P: P waves are inverted in inferior leads and buried in the tail end of the QRS (AVNRT) or present in the T waves (accessory pathway type).

Paroxysmal SVT: WPW and Tachycardia Mediated by an Accessory Pathway (AVRT)

Circus movement tachycardia (CMT), orthodromic reciprocating tachycardia (ORT), and AV reentrant tachycardia (AVRT) are all synonyms used to describe the most common type of SVT mediated by an accessory pathway. This type of paroxysmal SVT is usually initiated by a critically timed premature atrial of ventricular complex. The tachycardia loop propagates down the AV node and returns to the atrium via an accessory connection before returning back down the AV node. Since *the atrium and ventricle are activated sequentially*, P waves and QRS complexes are distinct from each other. Since retrograde pathway conduction is generally much more rapid than antegrade AV nodal conduction, *the retrograde P waves are inverted and separate from the QRS, usually found buried within the T wave.*

The majority of accessory pathways will only conduct in a single direction from the ventricle to the atrium. However, in about 25 % of patients with this type of tachycardia, the accessory pathway is capable of conduction in both directions. In those cases, pathway conduction is manifest on the resting ECG during sinus rhythm as a delta wave or "preexcitation." Individuals with both SVT and manifest preexcitation on their baseline ECG are said to have Wolff-Parkinson-White syndrome (WPW).

Very rarely, patients with WPW can have another type of AVRT known as "antidromic reciprocating tachycardia." In these cases, the arrhythmia propagates down the accessory pathway to the ventricle and then backwards up the AV node to reach the atrium. This produces a regular, wide QRS tachycardia.

Paroxysmal SVT: Atrioventricular Nodal Reentrant Tachycardia (AVNRT)

AVNRT is a reentrant arrhythmia that circles within the AV node or peri-AV nodal tissue. This arrhythmia is thought to occur when there are two extensions on the AV node (often referred to as "dual AV node pathways" or "dual AV node physiology"). The two AV nodal extensions generally have distinct conduction velocities and are referred to as the "fast pathway" and "slow pathway." The reentrant loop usually travels down the slow pathway and then turns up the fast pathway to complete the loop. The electrical signal branches

off to the ventricle at the same time that the retrograde fast pathway is activated. Since *the atrium and ventricle are activated simultaneously*, the P waves and QRS complexes overlap. Thus, *the retrograde P waves are inverted and buried within or "married" to the back of the preceding QRS complex with no separation between the two.*

PSVT recognition clues:

- Classically presents as palpitations that start and stop abruptly.
- Usually 200–300 bpm.
- Always regular, usually narrow QRS tachycardia.
- Wide QRS (bundle branch block or SVT with aberrancy) is sometimes observed.
- Typically initiated by a PAC or PVC (i.e., the first P wave to initiate tachycardia has morphology that is distinct from the subsequent P waves observed during sustained tachycardia).
- Bimodal age distribution: most commonly encountered in infants or adolescents but can be seen in any age group.
- Rarely associated with syncope.
- P waves are always inverted in the inferior leads (II, III, and AVF).
- AV block is not usually observed except upon tachycardia termination.
- Additional clues to differentiate ORT from AVNRT:
  - *ORT* has retrograde P waves that are inverted and distinct from the preceding QRS, usually buried within the T wave.
  - 25 % of those with *ORT* will have WPW in sinus rhythm.
  - *AVNRT* has retrograde P waves that are inverted and either concealed within the QRS complex or "married" to the back of it.
  - Patients with *AVNRT* do not usually have evidence of WPW in sinus rhythm, although a higher frequency of low atrial rhythm at baseline has been reported.

Other supraventricular arrhythmias:

Ectopic Atrial Tachycardia (EAT)

Ectopic atrial tachycardia (EAT) is an automatic tachycardia that originates from a discrete location in the right or left atrium, often in one of the atrial appendages or pulmonary veins. This is a uniquely pediatric arrhythmia, and its clinical presentation and natural course are distinct from the focal reentrant forms of atrial tachycardia commonly observed in adults. In contrast to the more common reentrant PSVT, this automatic arrhythmia cannot be terminated with vagal maneuvers or adenosine. EAT often occurs in short bursts, and while episodes of sustained tachycardia can certainly occur, 24-h Holter monitoring usually reveals frequent PACs, along with two- to four-beat runs of nonsustained EAT sprinkled throughout the monitoring period during the times that normal sinus rhythm predominates.

Rate: usually 180–240

Regularity: generally regular, although the rate may vary during "warm up" and "cooldown"

QRS: narrow

Relationship of QRS-P: P waves *precede* the QRS and tend to fall on the downslope of the T wave or after the T wave reaches baseline.

EAT recognition clues:

- A P wave usually precedes every QRS.
- The PR interval is slightly prolonged (160–200 ms).
- P wave morphology in tachycardia is distinctly different from P wave morphology in sinus rhythm, usually with a different P wave axis.
- EAT arising from the right atrial appendage, close to the sinus node, may share a similar axis with sinus P waves, but EAT P waves are usually more pointed and slightly abnormal appearing.
- Always regular, usually narrow QRS tachycardia.
- Wide QRS (bundle branch block or SVT with aberrancy) may be observed.
- AV block may be observed without tachycardia termination.
- A "warm-up" or "cooldown" phenomenon is sometimes observed as a gradual change in the P-P interval. The "warm-up" is particularly evident on the first few beats of tachycardia.
- EAT is not typically initiated by a PAC or PVC (i.e., the first P wave in tachycardia is identical in morphology to subsequent P waves).

Multifocal Atrial Tachycardia and Chaotic Tachycardia

Multifocal atrial tachycardia and chaotic tachycardia are other automatic arrhythmias that share many features with EAT. In contrast, these arrhythmias originate from multiple foci in the atrium. By definition, multifocal atrial tachycardia shows three distinct abnormal P wave morphologies on the ECG. These arrhythmias rarely occur in healthy children with no other medical issues, and they are much more commonly encountered in

infants with comorbid conditions like cardiomyopathies, postoperative atrial scars, or severe respiratory illness and/or pulmonary hypertension. These cannot usually be terminated by DC cardioversion or adenosine, and arrhythmia suppression with antiarrhythmic drugs is often difficult (Fig. 6.12).

The 4 R's of Multifocal Atrial Tachycardia and Chaotic Tachycardia

Rate: usually 220–300

Regularity: irregular

QRS: narrow (although wide QRS Ashman beats may be seen – similar to atrial fibrillation)

Relationship of QRS-P: P waves have multiple morphologies and *precede* the QRS.

Multifocal/chaotic atrial tachycardia recognition clues:

- Multiple P wave morphologies.
- Atrial and ventricular rhythms are both irregular.
- QRS is usually narrow, but wide QRS complexes can occur, particularly with short QRS coupling intervals (Ashman phenomenon).
- Atrial activity may occur in short "bursts" with frequent starting and stopping
- Usually does not respond to electrical cardioversion.

Atrial Fibrillation

Atrial fibrillation is the most disorganized of all the supraventricular tachycardias. The atria depolarize at very rapid rates, usually in the range of 300–500 bpm, and conduction to the ventricles is also irregular. This produces a characteristically "irregularly irregular" rhythm. In adults, atrial fibrillation is thought to be initiated from triggers within the pulmonary veins. In contrast, isolated atrial fibrillation is very rare in children with structurally normal hearts, and it much more commonly encountered in older children who have had surgery for congenital heart disease. More organized supraventricular arrhythmias like orthodromic reciprocating tachycardia and atrial flutter may degenerate into atrial fibrillation, and atrial fibrillation is

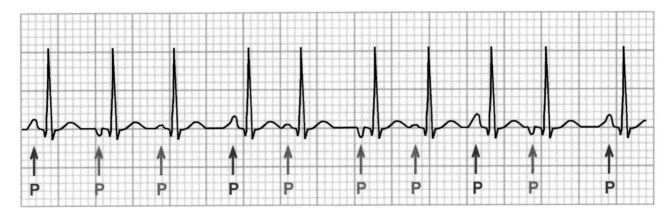

Fig. 6.12 A 32-year-old women, s/p atrial switch procedure with multifocal atrial tachycardia, note the three distinct appearing P waves

also more common in individuals with WPW pathways. On the ECG, atrial activity does not produce discreet P waves but rather irregular fluctuations from baseline that vary in size and shape.

Ashman phenomenon or Ashman beats are occasional wide QRS complexes seen during atrial fibrillation. These wide QRS beats usually follow a short R-R interval that is preceded by a long R-R interval. These beats, often mislabeled as PVCs, actually originate from above the AV node and represent aberrant conduction through the His-Purkinje system (Fig. 6.13).

The 4 R's of Atrial Fibrillation

Rate: ventricular rate is usually 150–250, atrial rate cannot be counted

Regularity: irregularly irregular

QRS: narrow (although wide QRS Ashman beats may be seen intermittently)

Relationship of QRS-P: distinct P waves are not seen

Atrial fibrillation recognition clues:

- There are no clear P waves; however, the baseline does wander with irregular deflections between QRS complexes.
- QRS rhythm is "irregularly irregular."
- QRS is usually narrow, but wide QRS complexes can occur, particularly with short QRS coupling intervals (Ashman phenomenon).
- Atrial fibrillation is usually a sustained arrhythmia, and sinus rhythm should resume when atrial fibrillation stops. Disorganized atrial activity that tends to occur in short "bursts" is more likely to be multifocal atrial tachycardia than traditional atrial fibrillation.
- Usually responds to electrical cardioversion.

Atrial Flutter

Atrial flutter is a reentrant arrhythmia occurring entirely within the atrium. Most commonly, the substrate for atrial flutter is an area of slow conduction in the floor of the right atrium known as the cavotricuspid isthmus. This "isthmus-dependent" flutter is usually encountered in structurally normal hearts, and the electrical wavefront travels in a circle around the right atrium. Counterclockwise circuits are called "typical flutter," and clockwise circuits are called "atypical flutter." Classic atrial flutter has an atrial rate of 300 bpm in adolescents and adults. In neonates, atrial rates are typically faster (350–450 bpm).

In patients with congenital heart disease, an even more atypical form of atrial flutter is often encountered in patients with atrial scarring resulting from surgical repair. This type of atrial flutter is referred to as intra-atrial reentrant tachycardia (IART). The atrial rate in these arrhythmias is generally much slower than in typical atrial flutter, with atrial rates of 200–300 bpm being common (Fig. 6.14).

The 4 R's of Atrial Flutter

Rate: atrial rate is usually 300 in adolescents and adults or 350–450 in neonates. Since 2:1 conduction is most common, the ventricular rate is usually 150–200.

Regularity: usually regular

QRS: narrow (although wide QRS Ashman beats may be seen intermittently, particularly if the rhythm is irregular)

Relationship of QRS-P: there is usually a fixed ratio of Ps to QRSs. P waves are often exactly halfway between QRS complexes (see Harold Bix rule).

Atrial flutter recognition clues:

- A characteristic "sawtooth" pattern can be seen throughout the ECG, particularly in the inferior leads.
- In classic "isthmus-dependent" atrial flutter, P waves are broad and continuous, with a sine wave appearance and no flat baseline between P waves. Unusual "intra-atrial reentrant tachycardias" encountered in patients after congenital heart surgery do not necessarily have this sine-wave appearance, and the P waves may be quite small.

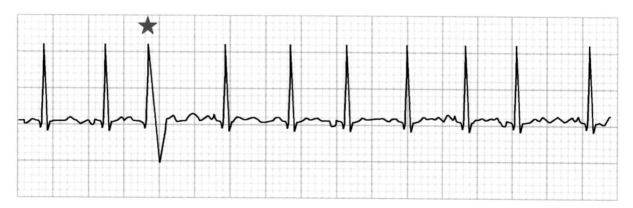

Fig. 6.13 Rapid atrial rate 300–400 bpm with irregular appearing P waves, variable AV block is noted with rapid and irregular ventricular rate. Note the wide QRS complex (*red star*); the PR interval is prolonged, and the RR interval is short preceding this wide QRS complex, which suggest Ashman phenomenon, rather than a PVC

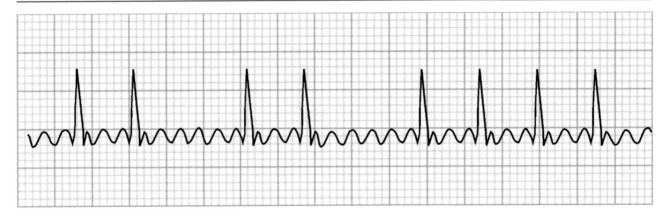

Fig. 6.14 Atrial flutter with variable AV block. P waves are well formed and regular with a rate of about 600 bpm. The ventricular rate is irregular, with a rate of about 140–160 bpm

- The QRS rhythm is usually regular with a fixed ratio of atrial to ventricular events (i.e., 2:1, 3:1, or 4:1 flutter).
- QRS is usually narrow. Ashman beats can occur with flutter, although that finding is much less common than in atrial fibrillation.
- Atrial flutter is usually a sustained arrhythmia, and sinus rhythm should resume when atrial flutter stops. Disorganized atrial activity that tends to occur in short "bursts" is more likely to be multifocal atrial tachycardia than traditional atrial fibrillation.
- Usually responds to electrical cardioversion.

The Harold Bix Rule: Harold Bix, a cardiologist from Vienna, noted that if the P wave is exactly halfway between two QRS complexes, there is a high likelihood that another P wave is buried inside the QRS. This finding is commonly observed in typical atrial flutter with 2:1 conduction, particularly when atrial rates are about 300 and ventricular rates are 150 bpm. The "hidden" P wave can be identified as a slurring in the upstroke or downstroke of the QRS.

Rhythms Arising from the Ventricles

Ventricular Extrasystoles or Premature Ventricular Contractions (PVCs)

PVCs are single depolarizations originating from the ventricles. The QRS is wide and distinctly different from the baseline narrow QRS seen in sinus rhythm. By themselves, PVCs are usually benign and many children with PVCs do not even have palpitations or any awareness of the fact that their heart is beating irregularly. Many systemic conditions and/or cardiomyopathies may cause PVCs. But in most cases, PVCs are idiopathic and no discernable cause can be identified.

A thorough workup for underlying electrolyte abnormalities or structural heart disease should be performed before deeming the problem benign. Antiarrhythmic drug ingestions should be considered, particularly in toddlers, and one should inquire about bottles of antiarrhythmic drugs in the household (Fig. 6.15).

PVC recognition clues:

- Always wide QRS.
- Not preceded by a premature p wave.
- PVC "fusion beats" may have only slight widening of the QRS if the beats occur immediately after the sinus P waves and fall into the normal PR interval.

Conditions that may cause PVCs:

- Electrolyte disturbances
- Misplaced central venous lines or intracardiac devices residing inside the ventricle
- Toxicity related to digoxin, antiarrhythmic drugs, or other medications
- Pericarditis and/or myocarditis
- Inotropic infusions (epinephrine, dopamine, etc.)
- Cardiomyopathies

PVCs are generally considered benign when:

- There is a uniform morphology (all PVCs appear identical).
- PVCs occur in isolation without couplets, triplets, or runs of ventricular tachycardia.
- The PVCs stop occurring once a certain heart rate threshold is reached during exercise.
- The heart is structurally and functionally normal by echocardiography.

Ventricular Escape Rhythms

These are slow, wide QRS rhythms that may emerge with profound slowing of the sinus node. These are usually benign. Slightly faster ventricular rhythms in the range of

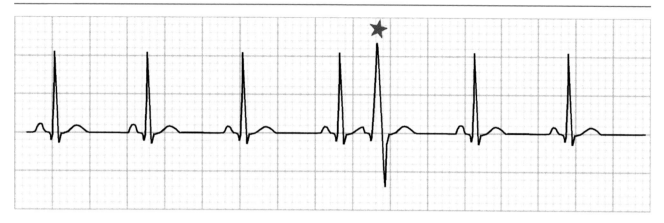

Fig. 6.15 Wide complex QRS (*red star*), occurring early and not precede by P wav suggesting premature ventricular contraction (PVC)

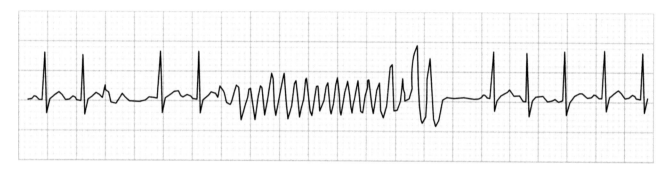

Fig. 6.16 VT may be polymorphic; note the different configuration of ventricular complexes. This tracing shows polymorphic VT (360 bpm) and is initiated by a PVC which falls on the preceding QRS-T vulnerable part of the T wave

60–100 bpm are generally referred to as "*accelerated ventricular rhythm*." While both are rare and technically abnormal, they are generally benign.

Ventricular Tachycardia (VT)

VT refers to an organized, rapid heart rhythm originating in the ventricles. The QRS is wide and the heart rhythm may be regular or irregular. PVCs may occur in couplets and triplets, but once there are four or more ventricular beats in a row, the definition of VT is met. *Monomorphic VT* refers to a ventricular tachycardia where each QRS complex is identical to the others and the rhythm is usually regular. *Polymorphic VT* refers to arrhythmias with multiple different QRS morphologies and an irregular rhythm.

There is a common perception that patients with VT are inherently more unstable than patients with SVT. This probably arises from the fact that VT in children is more commonly encountered in patients with underlying congenital heart disease or cardiac dysfunction. Also, very rapid VTs may deteriorate into ventricular fibrillation, causing cardiac arrest.

Despite the bad reputation that VT has earned, there are several forms of idiopathic VT that are actually quite benign. These are generally monomorphic and encountered in otherwise healthy children with structurally normal hearts. In this group, VT simply causes palpitations and may be indistinguishable from SVT by symptoms alone. Furthermore, since SVT can often occur with wide-QRS aberrancy, it may be difficult to differentiate VT from SVT on an ECG (Figs. 6.16, 6.17, and 6.18).

The prognosis in patients with VT often hinges on the underlying diagnosis, as patients with underlying chanelopathies (e.g. long QT syndrome) or cardiomyopathies have a higher liklihood of experiencing life-threatening cardiac arrest. For this reason, patients with VT require a thorough and comprehensive cardiac evaluation.

The 4 R's of Ventricular Tachycardia

Rate: usually 170–210 (generally VT is slower than SVT)

Regularity: monomorphic VT is usually regular, while polymorphic VT is irregular

QRS: always wide

Relationship of QRS-P: when P waves have no relation to QRS (VA dissociation), this is diagnostic; however, in patients with robust retrograde AV conduction, there may be inverted "retrograde p waves" buried in the upslope of the T waves.

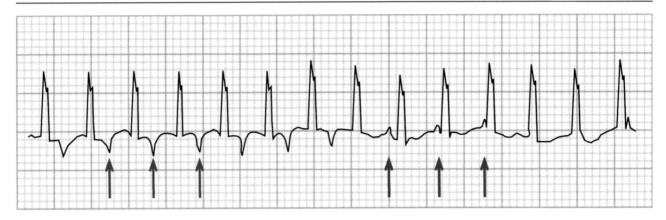

Fig. 6.17 Ventricular tachycardia without (*blue arrow*) and with (*red arrow*) VA dissociation

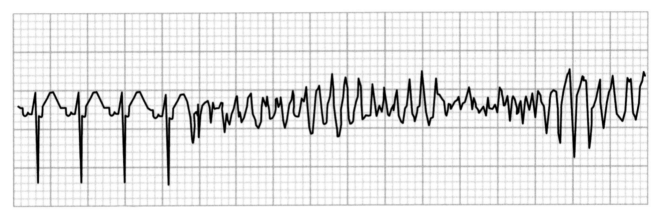

Fig. 6.18 Torsades de pointes (twisting of the points). The first 3 beats are sinus rhythm, followed by a PVC, then ventricular tachycardia with changing QRS axis

Ventricular Tachycardia Recognition Clues:

- Always wide QRS
- Rates are usually 170–210 bpm for monomorphic VT, but polymorphic VT may have rates exceeding 300 bpm.
- The following are pathognomonic for VT.
  - VA dissociation: P wave or atrial rate is slower than the ventricular rate.
  - Sinus capture or "fusion beats" are occasional narrow QRS beats that occur as the result of antegrade AV conduction during tachycardia
- Adenosine may help to demonstrate VA dissociation, but will not alter the ventricular rate or terminate tachycardia.

Ventricular Fibrillation

Ventricular fibrillation (VF) is a disorganized arrhythmia originating in the ventricles. The rhythm is usually sustained until cardioversion is performed, and patients are generally unconscious and pulseless within seconds of its commence-

ment. Low amplitude VF may be very fine and can be confused with asystole, particularly during a resuscitation where CPR or patient convulsions may perturb the ECG baseline. This distinction is critical to make because cardioversion, which is not indicated for asystole, is critical for patients with VF. When confusion arises, it may be helpful to briefly pause resuscitation efforts in order to record a 10–15 s rhythm strip, preferably with multiple leads. VF will show subtle variations in the electrogram amplitude, while asystole will be totally flat.

Ventricular fibrillation may also be confused with torsades de pointes, which is a very rapid type of polymorphic VT encountered in patients with long QT syndrome. Torsades often occur in short, nonsustained bursts and, by definition, follow sinus rhythm with a prolonged QT interval (Fig. 6.19).

Rhythms Arising from the AV Junction

Junctional rhythms may occur as benign junctional escape rhythms, accelerated junctional rhythm with intermediate heart rates, or as a fast tachyarrhythmia known as junctional accelerated tachycardia (JET).

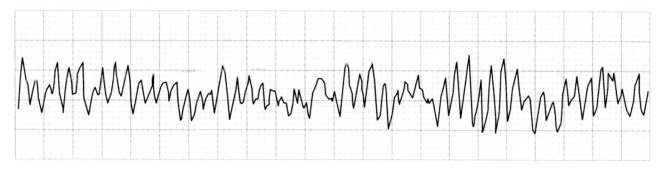

Fig. 6.19 Ventricular fibrillation

Conditions associated with junctional ectopic tachycardia (JET):

- Initial 24-h after surgery to repair congenital heart disease, particularly after surgery for large ventricular septal defects, tetralogy of Fallot, or AV canal defects
- Congenital JET – may be familial

The 4 R's of Junctional Ectopic Tachycardia

Rate: usually 150–220 bpm
Regularity: regular
QRS: narrow
Relationship of QRS-P: no relationship (when VA dissociation is present) or "retrograde P waves" falling on the upslope of the T wave

---

Junctional ectopic tachycardia recognition clues:

- QRS is narrow, although slight differences from the sinus QRS may be observed.
- In patients with fixed bundle branch blocks in sinus rhythm, the QRS morphology in JET should match that observed in sinus.
- JET is usually regular but may be irregular if sinus capture beats occur.
- There may be VA dissociation (this rules SVT out of the differential diagnosis).
- There may be inverted P waves if retrograde VA conduction is present.

Conclusions

While pediatric arrhythmias may be complex, a concise differential diagnosis can usually be made by rapidly identifying the rate, regularity, and QRS morphology.

With that in mind, careful examination of a 12-lead ECG usually helps to narrow the diagnosis. We end this chapter with a few helpful clinical pearls:

- Organized reentrant arrhythmias like atrial flutter, paroxysmal SVT, and monomorphic VT are generally very regular with few variations from beat to beat.
- Disorganized rhythms like atrial fibrillation, polymorphic VT, and multifocal atrial tachycardia are usually irregular.
- When differentiating wide QRS arrhythmias (VT vs. SVT with aberrancy), remember that SVT with aberrancy is generally much faster (220–280 bpm) than VT (170–210).
- In pediatric patients without congenital heart disease, 90 % of atrial flutter encountered is seen in the first 48 h of life. Outside of this window, regular narrow QRS tachycardia is adenosine-responsive paroxysmal SVT 90 % of the time.

References

1. Deal BJ. Supraventricular tachycardia mechanisms and natural history. In: Deal BJ, Wolff GS, Gelband H, editors. Current concepts in diagnosis and management of arrhythmias in infants and children. Armonk: Futura Publishing Company; 1998. p. 114–7.
2. Alexander ME. Ventricular arrhythmias in children and young adults. In: Walsh EP, Saul JP, Triedman JK, editors. Cardiac arrhythmias in children and young adults with congenital heart disease. Philadelphia: Lippincott Williams & Wilkins; 2001. p. 201–34.
3. Texter KM, Kertesz NJ, Friedman RA, Fenrich Jr AL. Atrial flutter in infants. J Am Coll Cardiol. 2006;48(5):1040–6.
4. Garson Jr A, Gillette PC, McNamara DG. Supraventricular tachycardia in children: clinical features, response to treatment, and long-term follow-up in 217 patients. J Pediatr. 1981;98:875–82.
5. Collins KK, Van Hare GF, Kertesz NJ, et al. Pediatric nonpostoperative junctional ectopic tachycardia medical management and interventional therapies. J Am Coll Cardiol. 2009;53(8):690–7.

Atrioventricular Conduction Abnormalities: Preexcitation, Heart Block, and Other Ventricular Conduction Abnormalities

William Bonney

Introduction

Each cardiac impulse originates in the sinus node with the ultimate objective of producing normal atrial and then ventricular contractions. Each heartbeat traverses the atrial tissue, AV node, bundle of His, and right and left bundle branches on the way to smaller branches in the His-Purkinje system and ultimately ventricular myocardium. Abnormalities in any of these structures produce varying degrees of atrioventricular conduction or heart block. While some of these disturbances may be nothing more than benign observations, others may be indicative of significant pathology that should be treated with pacing.

Normal AV Nodal Function

The AV node serves as a "relay station" directing atrial impulses to the bundle of His and then onto the right and left bundle branches. When functioning appropriately, the left and right ventricles contract synchronously and efficiently. Normally, the ventricular septum is activated first, just milliseconds before right and left ventricular contraction occur simultaneously. This produces small "septal Q waves" on the ECG which are best seen in the inferior and lateral leads. In healthy hearts, this entire process takes place in less than a tenth of a second, and consequently, the QRS is narrow. The AV node is located anteriorly and superiorly, and hence, the normal QRS axis is inferior. Since the left ventricle is more massive than the right ventricle, the predominant ECG forces are leftward and posterior when the two ventricles contract together.

W. Bonney, MD
Department of Cardiology, Children's Hospital of Philadelphia,
34th Street and Civic Center Boulevard,
Philadelphia, PA 19104, USA
e-mail: BONNEYW@email.chop.edu

Left and Right Bundle Branch Block (LBBB and RBBB)

When bundle branch block occurs, one of the ventricles will not be depolarized through the His-Purkinje system. Instead, the electrical wave front travels quickly through the bundle branch which is intact, resulting in rapid depolarization of the ipsilateral ventricle, and then depolarization drifts slowly over the contralateral ventricle from cell to cell. Hence, the ventricles depolarize sequentially rather than simultaneously, and the resulting QRS is prolonged and wide. The initial QRS deflection may be narrow as His-Purkinje conduction predominates, and the terminal QRS is slurred as slower conduction occurs from cell to cell through the second ventricle (Figs. 7.1 and 7.2).

It is important to remember that when right or left bundle branch block is present, the ECG becomes useless as a tool to assess for right or left ventricular hypertrophy. When consulting a reference table that lists upper limits of normal for R wave and S wave voltages, one must remember that these voltages represent the combined electrical output resulting from left and right ventricles contracting at the same time. Trying to decide which ventricle is enlarged in the presence of bundle branch block would be analogous to staging a tug-of-war match in which one team gets a 10-s head start before the other team is allowed to start pulling on the rope.

Right Bundle Branch Block

While full-blown right bundle branch block is uncommon in children with structurally normal hearts, incomplete right bundle branch block and subtle right ventricular conduction delays are not that uncommon. An RSR′ pattern may be observed in lead V1 up to 10 % of normal children. When interpreting ECGs, it is important to make a distinction between RSR′ with an entirely narrow QRS, which is normal, and RSR′ patterns with a wide QRS, which may be abnormal (Fig. 7.3). The terms "incomplete right bundle branch block" and "right ventricular conduction delay"

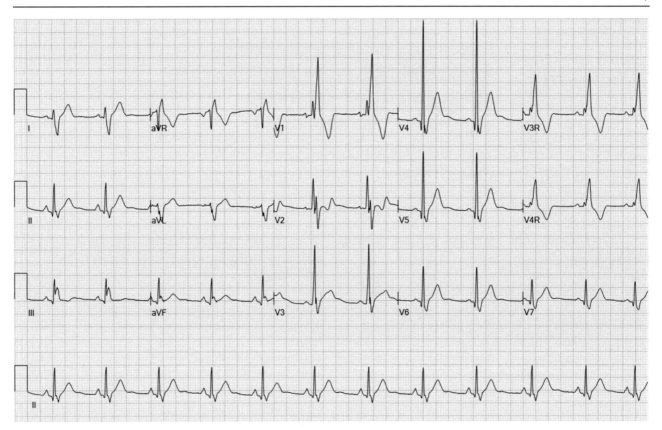

Fig. 7.1 Right bundle branch block. The QRS complex is wide = 160 ms. Note the RSR′ pattern of QRS in the right chest lead (V1); the terminal R′ is much wider than the initial R wave. S wave in the left chest lead is slurred

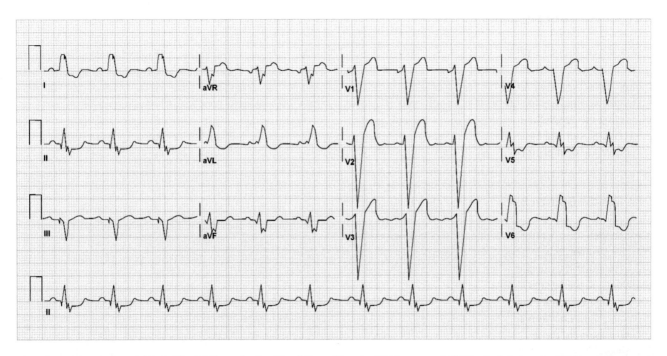

Fig. 7.2 Left bundle branch block. The QRS complex is wide = 160 ms. Note the RSR′ pattern of QRS in the left chest lead (V6) and the slurred S wave in the right chest lead

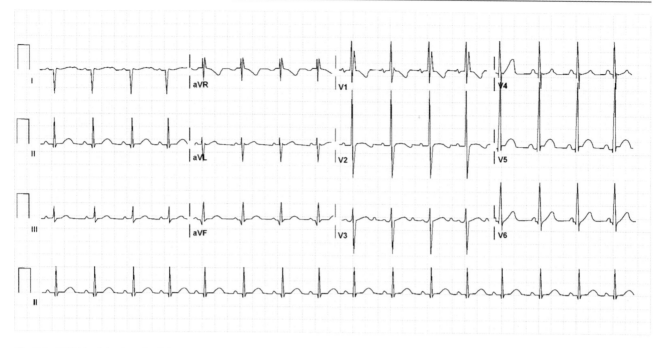

Fig. 7.3 RSR′ in right chest lead (V1) without widening of the QRS duration (80 ms). This is a normal finding in children. This suggests normal conduction through the bundles of His

should be reserved for those with a QRS duration that is slightly prolonged, but not enough to meet the criteria for full-blown right bundle branch block.

Criteria for Right Bundle Branch Block

1. QRS is prolonged >120 ms (above the upper limit of normal for age) with normal activation during the first half (approximately 60 ms) of the QRS complex.
2. Right axis deviation, especially for the slurred terminal portion of the QRS.
3. Terminal slurring of the QRS is rightward (S wave in I and V6) and anterior (R wave in V1).

Left Bundle Branch Block

The spontaneous occurrence of complete LBBB in children is rare. Most often, this is observed in children with cardiomyopathy or other disease of the left ventricle or as a consequence of damage to the left bundle branch during surgery. When the cardiac impulse cannot traverse the left bundle branch, it travels to the right bundle branch and then through the interventricular septum to the left ventricle. Consequently, the septum is activated in reverse direction from right to left. Hence, the typical "septal Q waves" observed in inferior and lateral leads are absent. In the right precordial leads, the usual initial R wave is gone and there is a QS pattern instead (Fig. 7.2).

Criteria for Left Bundle Branch Block

1. QRS is prolonged >120 ms (above the upper limit of normal for age).
2. Left axis deviation for the patient's age.
3. The slurred QRS complex is directed to the left and posteriorly.
   (a) Absent Q waves and slurred broad R waves in leads I, aVL, and V6
   (b) rS or QS deflection in leads V1 and V2
4. ST- and T-wave vector 180° discordant to the QRS vector.

Heart Block

Heart block in children can be congenital or acquired. There are three degrees of heart block, and individuals will commonly display one or more degrees of block throughout the day depending on extrinsic factors like activity, vagal tone, and catecholamine state.

First-Degree AV Block

The term "first-degree AV block" is somewhat of a misnomer because every atrial beat conducts to the ventricle; hence AV conduction is *delayed* but there is no real AV *block*. Regardless, the term is commonly used and accepted (Fig. 7.4).

Recognition Clues

- A P wave precedes every QRS and a QRS follows every P wave.
- The PR interval exceeds the upper limit of normal for age and rate (see Appendix).

Anything producing conduction delay between the atrium and the ventricle will prolong the PR interval. The most common cause is increased vagal tone. Conduction delay in the His-Purkinje system after heart surgery may prolong the PR interval as well. The PR may also be prolonged in rheumatic fever or Kawasaki disease. Mild degrees of first-degree AV block are generally benign and require no treatment.

Second-Degree AV Block

In first-degree heart block, all of the P waves conduct, and in third-degree heart block, none of the P waves conduct. Second-degree block, therefore, describes the various

bradyarrhythmias that display AV conduction on *some* of the beats but not *all* of the beats. There are four types of second-degree AV block, described below.

- Mobitz I
- Mobitz II
- 2:1 AV block
- High-grade AV block

Second-Degree AV Block: Type I or Mobitz I (Wenckebach)

In Wenckebach conduction, the PR interval gradually prolongs before finally there is a P wave that is not followed by a QRS. The PR interval shortens on the beat following AV block, gradually prolonging again on subsequent beats as the cycle repeats. This can be a normal finding and is often observed in athletes during sleep. During invasive EP testing, virtually every individual's AV node has an upper limit of conduction, and Wenckebach phenomenon is observed at this upper limit (Fig. 7.5).

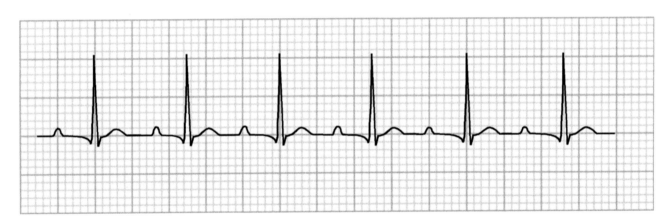

Fig. 7.4 First-degree AV block. Note the PR interval is prolonged, measuring 200 ms; normal in children less than 16 years of age is 80–180 ms

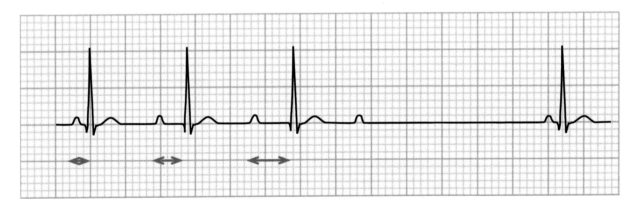

Fig. 7.5 Second-degree heart block, Mobitz type I (Wenckebach). The PR interval lengthens with each beat and on the 4th beat in this example the P wave is not conducted

Mobitz I, Second-Degree AV Block Recognition Clues

- This is an *irregular* rhythm.
- Gradual prolonging of the PR interval until finally a P wave does not conduct.
- The R-R interval between subsequent beats shortens as the PR interval prolongs.

Causes: increased vagal tone, anti-arrhythmic drugs or digoxin and secondary to injury to the AV node after surgery for congenital heart disease.

Management: This is generally a benign finding that does not require intervention in the absence of symptoms. It is particularly common in well-trained endurance athletes. Rarely, in symptomatic individuals temporary or permanent pacing may be required.

Second-Degree AV Block: Type II or Mobitz II

Type II AV block does not display any gradual prolonging of the PR interval prior to AV block; rather, the PR interval remains the same and intermittently sinus beats are not conducted. Mobitz II, in contrast with Wenckebach conduction, is considered an abnormal finding.

Recognition Clues

- This is an *irregular* rhythm.
- The PR interval on conducted beats remains constant.

Mobitz II block is often related to conduction system disease below the level of the AV node in the His bundle or the bundle branches. Symptomatic bradycardia with second-degree heart block is an indication for temporary or permanent pacing. In asymptomatic infants who have undergone surgery for congenital heart disease, second-degree heart block is an indication for pacing.

- *Note: In otherwise healthy children who have not had heart surgery, Mobitz II AV block is extremely rare. However, Mobitz I AV block may display only a subtle prolongation of the PR interval prior to eventual block. The best way to identify PR interval prolongation is to compare the* last beat before block *with the* first beat after conduction returns.

Second-Degree AV Block: 2:1 AV Block

Definition: In two-to-one AV block, every other atrial beat does not conduct. Since there is never more than one conducted beat in a row, there is no opportunity to look for gradual prolongation of the PR interval, and hence, 2:1 AV block may represent Mobitz I or Mobitz II block. In 2:1 AV block, the etiology is similar as Mobitz I or Mobitz II block. Patients with both Mobitz I and Mobitz II block can display 2:1 AV block at times (Fig. 7.6).

Recognition Clues

- This is a *regular* rhythm.
- The PR interval on conducted beats usually remains constant.

Second-Degree AV Block: High-Grade AV Block

The term "high-grade AV block" applies to the patient with nearly complete heart block but clear evidence of occasional conduction. Temporary or permanent pacing may be indicated in symptomatic individuals (Fig. 7.7).

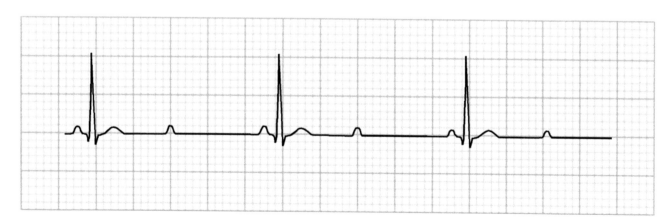

Fig. 7.6 Second-degree AV block Mobitz type II with 2:1 block

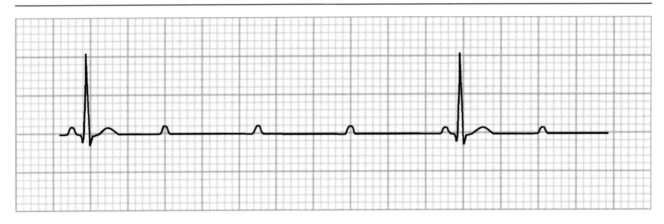

Fig. 7.7 Second-degree AV block: High-grade AV block. Note that there are three non-conducted P waves in a row

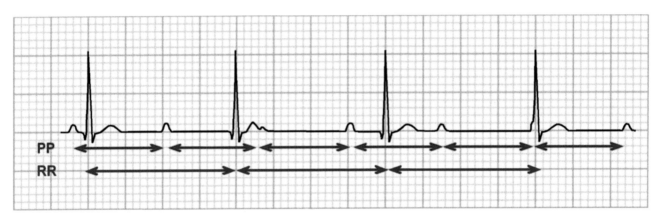

Fig. 7.8 Third-degree AV block. Note the regular P (atrial) and ventricular (QRS) rates. However, there is no synchrony between the P and QRS waves. The atrial rate is faster than the ventricular rate (PP interval (*red arrow*) is = 120/min, while RR interval (*blue arrow*) is = 75/min)

Recognition Clues

- Two or more P waves in a row are not followed by a QRS.
- Appears similar to complete heart block except occasional atrial beats have AV conduction.

Third-Degree AV Block

Complete heart block can be congenital or acquired and is caused by conduction block at the level of the AV node, His bundle, or Purkinje conduction system. In some instances congenital complete heart block is caused by maternal lupus, although many mothers of infants with congenital heart block have no evidence of autoimmune disease. Complete heart block in children is often the unintended consequence of surgery to repair congenital heart disease, particularly after repair of large ventricular septal defects, tetralogy of Fallot, or AV canal defects. Other acquired causes of heart block include Lyme disease (first-, second-, or third-degree heart block are

possible), cardiomyopathy, and anti-arrhythmic drug overdose. Myocardial infarction can cause heart block because of ischemia to the AV node or His-Purkinje system (Fig. 7.8).

Recognition Clues

- The QRS rate should be *regular* in complete heart block. The atrial rate is also usually regular. Any irregularity in the ventricular rate should raise suspicion for intermittent AV conduction (second-degree block).
- It is impossible to diagnose complete heart block unless there are more P waves than QRS complexes. For example, in a patient with a sinus rate of 60 bpm and accelerated junctional rhythm at 80 bpm, AV conduction cannot be evaluated because the ventricular rate is "outrunning" the atrial rate.
- QRS morphology depends on the escape rhythm in complete heart block. Most patients will have a junctional escape rhythm with regular, narrow QRS complexes. Patients with a ventricular escape rhythm will have wide QRS morphology.

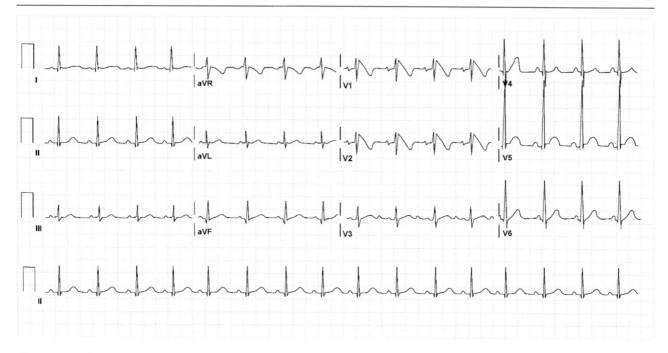

Fig. 7.9 Brugada syndrome. Note the RSR′ pattern in right chest leads (V1 & V2) with coved ST elevation

Brugada Syndrome

With an incidence of 1:20,000 individuals, Brugada syndrome is extremely rare. Even among individuals with this disease, the ECG may not always display the classic "type I" pattern that is diagnostic of this disease. However, Brugada syndrome remains an important cause of sudden death in young people. It is imperative for practitioners to have some familiarity with this pattern, particularly for the purposes of ECG screening for the evaluation of syncope and other suspected arrhythmias. To further confuse the issue, incomplete right bundle branch block is very common and when certain features are present, variations of RBBB and incomplete RBBB can look strikingly similar to the Brugada pattern (Figs. 7.9, 7.10, 7.11, and 7.12).

Type I Brugada syndrome manifests as coved ST segment in leads V1 and V2. Type II on the other hand manifests as saddleback ST segment in right chest leads. These findings, in either type, may or may not be associated with RSR′ pattern of QRS in right chest leads.

Hemiblocks or Fascicular Blocks

The left and right bundle branches as they traverse the ventricles go on to further divide into several divisions or fascicles. The left bundle branches into three divisions (septal, anterior-superior, and posterior-inferior). Block of either the anterior-superior division or posterior-inferior division is referred to as "hemiblock."

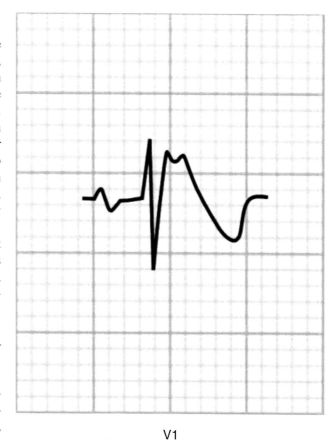

V1

Fig. 7.10 Brugada syndrome type II; note the saddleback appearance of ST segment in lead V1

Fig. 7.11 Both Brugada and incomplete RBBB ECGs show an RSR′ pattern in V1 and V2 with a narrow R segment and a wide R′ segment. However, RBBB ECGs show terminal slurring of the QRS in lateral leads (I, V6), while this is not typical of Brugada. Also, the ST segment has a convex curve in RBBB, while the Brugada ECG is flat or concave

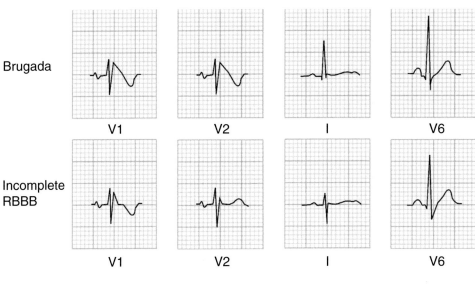

Fig. 7.12 An RSR′ pattern with wide QRS. The terminal R′ portion may raise concern for Brugada disease. One helpful way to differentiate the rare Brugada pattern from the relatively common incomplete RBBB pattern is to examine the ST segment. In type I Brugada, this segment is "coved" or convex, and the dashed line is bent outward. In right bundle branch block, the ST segment is convex with the dashed line bent inward

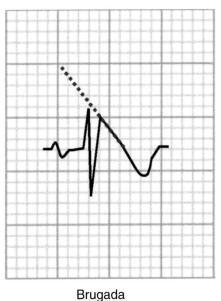 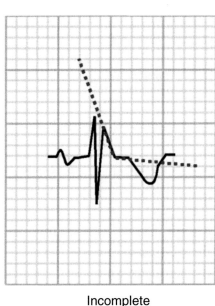

Block in the anterior division produces a marked left axis deviation since the superior and anterior portion is the LV is the last to depolarize. In children, this pattern is commonly observed in patients with certain congenital heart diseases (i.e., complete atrioventricular canal or tricuspid atresia) (Fig. 7.13).

When the posterior division is blocked, there is right axis deviation as the wave front is directed inferiorly and to the right. This is extremely rare in children.

Nonspecific Interventricular Block

When the QRS is clearly prolonged but specific criteria for LBBB or RBBB are not met, the terms "nonspecific interventricular block" or "interventricular conduction delay" can be applied. These are frequently observed in pediatric patients with complex congenital heart disease after surgery, especially in the single-ventricle population (Fig. 7.14).

Preexcitation (WPW)

Normally, the AV node is the only electrical connection between the top and bottom chambers of the heart, as the atria and ventricles are otherwise electrically insulated from one another. In a normal ECG, there is almost always some flat line segment in the PR interval between the end of the P wave and the beginning of the QRS complex. Preexcitation exists when all or some part of the ventricular muscle is activated prematurely by the atrial impulse. In these cases, the prematurely activated areas

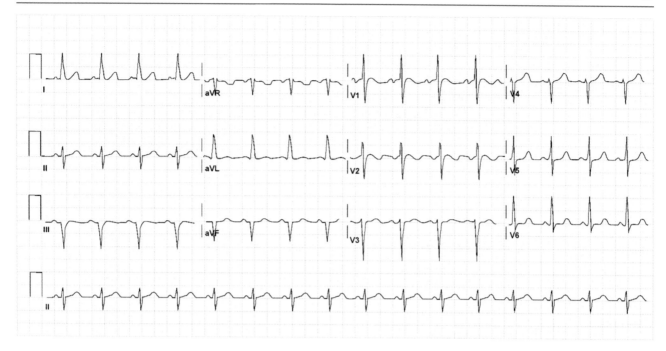

Fig. 7.13 Complete AVC defect. Block in the anterior division produces a marked left axis deviation since the superior and anterior portion in the LV is the last to depolarize

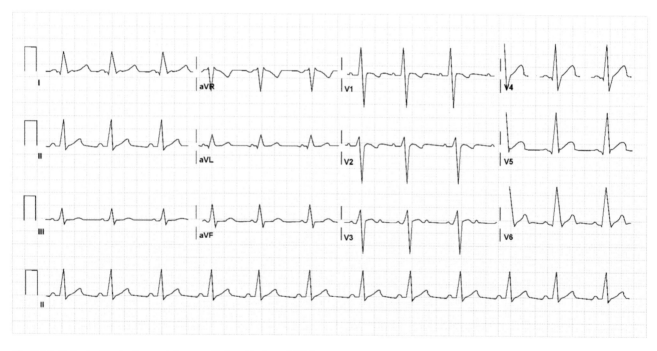

Fig. 7.14 Patient with single ventricle; note slight widening of QRS complex without typical features of right or left bundle branch block

depolarize sooner than what would be expected if the impulse reached the ventricles only by way of the normal atrioventricular conduction system. Consequently, there is a subtle upward slurring of the QRS (delta wave) and the flat, isoelectric portion of the PR segment is eliminated (Fig. 7.15).

Atrioventricular bypass tracts or "accessory pathways" account for the vast majority of preexcited ECGs. These accessory pathways, also known as Kent fibers, are essentially direct electrical connections between the atria and ventricles that circumvent the normal AV node and His-Purkinje system. Each accessory pathway has its own unique properties and conduction characteristics and the QRS pattern may look very different depending on where the pathway exists within the heart.

Fig. 7.15 Diagram illustrating mechanism of WPW. One way of understanding how WPW works is to think of a road intersection. In a normal intersection, if you want to turn right, you have to go up to the traffic light (AV node) make a complete stop, pause, and then turn. In the case of WPW, there is an extra ramp (accessory pathway) that allows you to turn right past a yield sign without stopping. A visual hint is the similarity between the appearance of a delta wave on ECG and the road ramp on this map

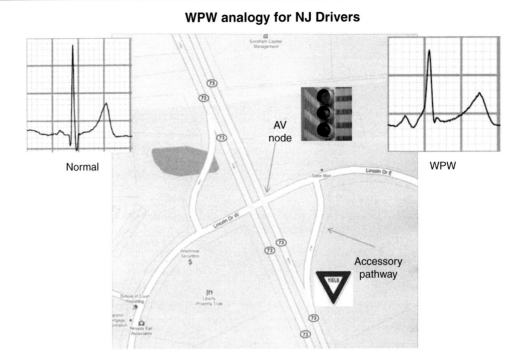

Accessory pathways may be unidirectional or bidirectional in nature. Those capable of conduction in the forward direction (atria to ventricles) produce the classic delta wave on ECG. Pathways that conduct in the retrograde direction (ventricle to atria) are usually associated with supraventricular tachycardia and symptoms of palpitations. Electrophysiology purists state that in order to use the term "Wolff-Parkinson-White *syndrome*" one must demonstrate both findings of SVT and evidence of preexcitation on the ECG in sinus rhythm. However, most practical cardiologists apply the diagnosis of "Wolff-Parkinson-White" to all patients with clear evidence of a delta wave regardless of symptoms. Patients with unidirectional accessory pathways conducting only in the retrograde direction may have SVT, but their ECGs in sinus rhythm are normal. These patients are said to have "concealed accessory pathways" and it would be erroneous to use the term WPW in them.

The classic ECG findings in WPW are a short PR interval and a prolonged QRS with a slurred QRS upstroke. Some pathways, particularly those on the right side of the heart, tend to produce more profound QRS prolongation and more obvious preexcitation. Left-sided pathways tend to produce more subtle findings. Nonetheless, once the diagnosis of WPW is confirmed, the clinical course and risk of arrhythmias is the same regardless of how the ECG looks. Just as a

woman can't be "just a little bit pregnant," a child cannot be "a little bit preexcited" (Figs. 7.16 and 7.17).

There are no strict criteria for diagnosing WPW on an ECG. In general, the PR interval is short and the QRS is prolonged, but the absolute measurements of those intervals do not always fall outside the upper and lower limits of normal. It must be emphasized that the short PR and prolonged QRS of WPW are more of a *qualitative* than a *quantitative* assessment.

Absence of septal Q waves in the inferior and/or lateral leads is one clue to the presence of preexcitation, and this is seen in up to 85 % of patients with WPW. This is not diagnostic, however, as up to 20 % of normal patients will have absent septal Q waves.

Absence of the delta wave during SVT is another important finding in patients with WPW. The most common form of SVT seen in patients with WPW is orthodromic reciprocating tachycardia. In this arrhythmia, the electrical wave front travels from the atria to the ventricles via the normal AV node and His-Purkinje system and then returns to the atrium via retrograde conduction through the accessory pathway. Since there is no pathway conduction in the anterograde direction, the QRS is not prolonged until SVT stops and sinus rhythm resumes (Figs. 7.18 and 7.19).

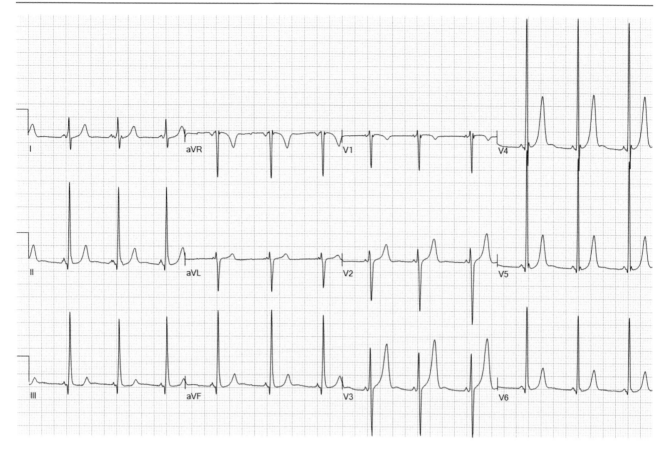

Fig. 7.16 Example of a short PR and slightly slurred QRS in a patient *without* WPW. While there is a subtle upslurring of the QRS in leads I and V1, there is actually a small, flat, isoelectric line between the end of the P wave and the beginning of the QRS in leads II, III, V5, and V6. In addition, septal Q waves are visible in the inferior and lateral leads

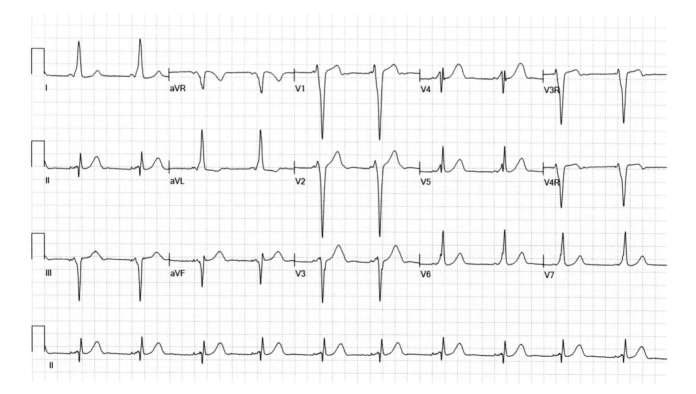

Fig. 7.17 WPW with clear preexcitation in a patient with a right-sided accessory pathway. The QRS is clearly prolonged, more so at the base than at the apex of the QRS. The PR interval is short in every lead with virtually no flat isoelectric segment in the PR interval

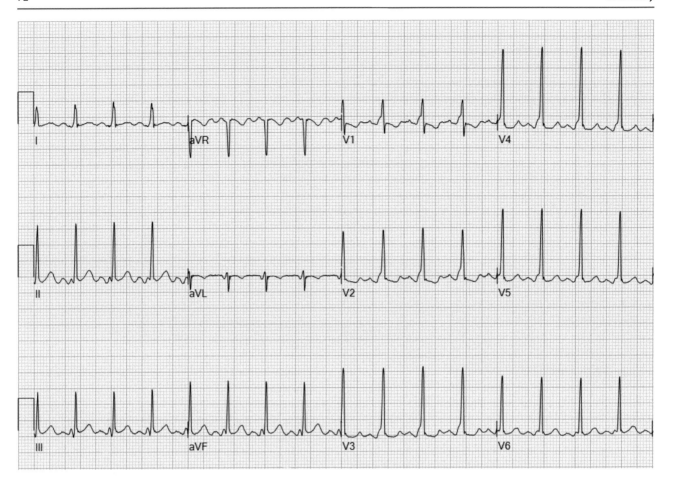

Fig. 7.18 Subtle preexcitation in a patient with a left-sided WPW pathway. While the QRS appears narrow in some leads (II, III, aVF), it is clearly wide at the base in others (V1, V2, V4, V5). Also, the QRS upstroke begins immediately at the end of the p wave without any flat isoelectric line in the PR

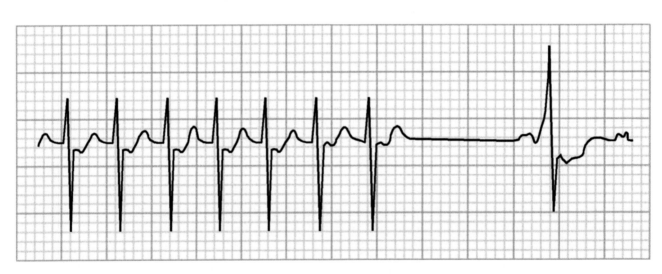

Fig. 7.19 The QRS is narrow during SVT. The delta wave is evident when SVT stops and sinus rhythm resumes

Further Reading

1. Durrer D, Schuilenburg RM, Wellens HJ. Preexcitation revisited. Am J Cardiol. 1970;25:690–7.
2. Heller J, Hagege AA, Besse B, et al. "Crochetage" (notch) on R wave in inferior limb leads: a new independent electrocardiographic sign of atrial septal defect. J Am Coll Cardiol. 1996;27(4):877–82.
3. Josephson M. Chapter 5. Intraventricular conduction disturbances. In: Josephson ME, editor. Clinical cardiac electrophysiology, techniques and interpretations. Philadelphia: Wolters Kluwer, Lippincott Williams & Wilkins, 2008.
4. Liberman L, Pass R, Starc T, et al. Uncovering the septal Q wave and other electrocardiographic changes in pediatric patients with pre-excitation before and after ablation. Am J Cardiol. 2010;105(2):214–6.

Cardiac Ischemia, Injury, and Infarction

8

Shaun Mohan and William Bonney

The ECG has been an irreplaceable diagnostic test in the evaluation of suspected myocardial injury. While children with structurally normal hearts are far less likely than adults to have acute coronary syndromes or true ischemic injury, it is not unusual for a child to present with chest pain in a setting that cardiac ischemia needs to be ruled out. Along with a careful history and exam, an ECG is an essential part of the workup for a child with acute chest pain. In otherwise healthy children without a history of congenital heart disease or cardiomyopathy, cardiac ischemia is exceedingly rare. However, it is not that uncommon to encounter benign forms of ST elevation and other T wave changes on an ECG. The aim of this chapter is to sort out true electrocardiographic patterns of ischemia from benign incidental findings.

It is important to note that there are a handful of conditions in the pediatric population with the probability of acute myocardial injury (Table 8.1). In this group of patients, an ECG is very helpful in making the diagnosis of ischemia, injury, or infarction, particularly if the child is able to adequately describe their chest pain. An ECG is also helpful in the cardiac intensive care unit for certain congenital heart diseases in the acute postoperative period, especially when there are signs of hemodynamic compromise or low cardiac output.

Interpreting ST and T wave changes in children who have undergone surgery for congenital heart disease can be challenging. Whenever possible, an ECG obtained in a child complaining of chest pain or symptoms suggestive of cardiac pathology should be compared to a prior ECG. An understanding of what constitutes pathologic T waves, ST-T wave changes, and pathologic Q waves requires appreciating the normal patterns and age-related changes that occur in an ECG as a child progresses from infancy to adolescence and finally adulthood.

When obtaining the history in a child or adolescent with chest pain, who has a structurally normal heart, one should consistently inquire about the use of illegal substances. Illegal substances can increase the risk of coronary vasospasm and precipitate myocardial ischemia, such as with cocaine.

In adults, ECG patterns that herald myocardial ischemia, injury, and infarction are well described, and there are clearly published guidelines on ECG standards and interpretation [1, 2]. The ECG criteria in children for myocardial injury are less specific, owing to the age-related changes that occur in a pediatric ECG. The accepted criteria among pediatric cardiologists can be traced to a postmortem study of autopsy-proved cases of transmural myocardial infarction and electrocardiographic evidence of myocardial infarction [3]. This study helps to form the basis for defining myocardial infarction in children in the absence of larger retrospective studies.

Evaluating ischemia or infarction on a 12-lead ECG requires revisiting certain concepts in electrocardiography. Diagnosis of ischemia requires that ST elevation be present in two or more contiguous leads [1–4]. The phrase "contiguous leads" refers to the precordial and limb leads referencing anatomic areas of the heart that are supplied by the coronary arteries. Any two leads that represent similar anatomic areas of the heart (assuming normal levocardia and ventricular looping) are considered contiguous (Table 8.2). For example, ST elevation in both leads I and aVL would be a more specific finding than ST elevation in either one of those leads alone or in leads I and V1 (not contiguous leads).

S. Mohan, MD, MPH
Department of Cardiology, Section of Electrophysiology,
Texas Children's Hospital, 6621 Fannin Street,
MC 1934C, Houston, TX 77030, USA
e-mail: shaun.mohan@bcm.edu

W. Bonney, MD (✉)
Department of Cardiology, Children's Hospital of Philadelphia,
34th Street and Civic Center Boulevard,
Philadelphia, PA 19104, USA
e-mail: BONNEYW@email.chop.edu

© Springer International Publishing Switzerland 2016
R. Abdulla et al. (eds.), *Pediatric Electrocardiography: An Algorithmic Approach to Interpretation*,
DOI 10.1007/978-3-319-26258-1_8

Table 8.1 Conditions which may be associated with myocardial ischemia

Category	Lesions
Congenital coronary anomalies	Anomalous origin of the coronary artery ALCAPA (anomalous coronary artery from the pulmonary artery) Coronary ostial atresia (particularly in Williams syndrome)
Congenital heart disease repair/palliation	D-TGA status post arterial switch operation Ross operation for aortic stenosis or critical AS Pulmonary atresia with intact ventricular septum with RV-dependent coronary circulation Any surgical procedure involving manipulation of the coronary arteries
Cardiomyopathies	Myocarditis Dilated cardiomyopathy Hypertrophic cardiomyopathy Coronary vasculopathy status post heart transplant
Extracardiac disease	Vasculitides (systemic lupus erythematosus, Takayasu's arteritis) Kawasaki's disease Sickle cell anemia Familial hypercholesterolemia Thrombophilias Drug ingestion (i.e., cocaine)

Table 8.2 Ischemia localization in the 12-lead ECG

Anatomic localization	Coronary artery distribution	Frontal leads (limb leads)	Horizontal (precordial leads)
Lateral	Proximal left anterior descending artery (LAD)	aVL, I	V5, V6
Anterior	LAD after first diagonal branch		V1, V2, V3
Anterolateral	Proximal LAD	aVL, I	V1, V2, V3, V4, V5, V6
Inferior	Right main coronary artery (RCA)	II, III, aVF	
Posterior	Posterior descending artery (PDA)		V1, V2

Table 8.3 Changes in ECG manifestation of cardiac ischemia over time

Early ischemia (few hours)	Inverted T waves
Hyperacute phase (few hours)	Elevated ST segments +/− deep and wide Q waves
Early evolving phase (a few days)	Deep and wide Q waves with continued ST elevation and T wave changes
Late evolving phase (2–3 weeks)	Deep and wide Q waves, sharply inverted T waves
Resolving phase (years)	Deep and wide Q waves with almost normal T waves

Determination of ischemic changes on an ECG requires analysis of all leads to detect anatomic patterns of injury corresponding to specific distribution of coronary blood flow. However, one should keep in mind that diffuse ischemic changes in all leads may be apparent if a global ischemic process was taking place as in myocarditis, pericarditis, cardiomyopathy, or significant hypotensive shock. When evaluating an ECG, it is important to proceed in a systematic order so as to not miss other potential abnormalities.

The ST segment is the part of the ECG that must be evaluated when determining if an ischemic pattern of injury is taking place. The ST segment is the quiet phase after the QRS (representing ventricular depolarization) and before the T wave (ventricular repolarization). The changes that may occur include ST segment shifts (elevation or depression), changes in the amplitude or vector of the T wave, and lengthening or shortening of the ST segment duration.

When myocardial injury takes place, there is a predictable sequence of changes that occur in an ECG (Table 8.3). These changes may be global if a generalized process occurs in the setting of hypotensive shock from a cardiac arrest or in contiguous leads if specific coronary artery distribution is the culprit. As a region of myocardium becomes necrotic, there is a surrounding area of injury and this is further surrounded by a zone of ischemia. Each ECG lead records a vector of conduction as the action potential propagates through the myocardium. If an area of myocardium is necrotic, electricity will not traverse that region of injury; in fact, the initial vector of conduction will point away from the contiguous leads, as represented by a pathologic Q wave. If these pathologic Q waves occur in a specific anatomic distribution, then infarction of tissue may have already occurred. The key is to recognize ischemic injury before these pathologic Q waves have manifested.

ECG changes due to acute myocardial infarction are time dependent. A careful history for a child or adolescent who is

able to characterize the pain (particularly the onset and duration of pain) will help determine onset of disease and as such
allow detection of specific ECG changes. In the acute setting, ST changes and pathologic Q waves are pathognomonic
signs for infarction on an ECG. In adults, the terms Q-wave
vs non-Q-wave infarction may be used. A Q wave typically
represents transmural involvement of the myocardium.
When the ischemia/infarction is limited to the subendocardium, Q waves may not manifest and instead ST depression
(with or without T wave changes) will be apparent on an
ECG. The ECG is more sensitive for classic transmural
infarctions than for more subtle subendocardial injury.
Again, clinical findings that enhance the pre-test probability
like cardiac biomarkers (troponin, CK-MB) and clinical
characteristics often help in making the correct diagnosis.

It is worth mentioning the term "peri-infarction block."
This is a pattern on an ECG that is often seen in the antero-
lateral and inferior leads when there is transmural infarction.
This is a pattern where the terminal QRS vector is directed
toward the area of infarction in addition to a pathologic Q
wave. The "block" term refers to involvement of one of the
fascicles (right bundle, septal, left anterior or posterior fas-
cicle) in the infarct, and consequently the area distal to the
infarct will depolarize later than intact myocardium.

Benign Variants Which May Be Confused with Ischemic Changes

T Waves

As mentioned above, T wave changes may be the initial ECG
manifestation of ischemia. Therefore, familiarity with the normal pattern of the T wave in the pediatric population will allow
identifying such features as a normal finding in certain age
groups rather than indicative of pathology, such as ischemia.
The T wave presents the average vector of ventricular repolarization. In adults, the T wave vector is directed toward the left in
the precordial leads (horizontal plane). Conversely in children,
the T wave is anterior (as represented by an upright T wave in
V1) in the postnatal period and becomes more posterior by the
end of the first week of life (with a resultant negative T wave in
V1). The T wave vector remains in this position for the first
5–10 years of life and sometimes even well into late adolescence (particularly in athletes). For the majority of children after
the age of 10 years, the T vector becomes progressively more
anterior and leftward. These changes are important to bear in
mind if the patient is an adolescent or younger child complaining of chest pain. Normally, the T wave vector is oriented toward
the left with upright T waves in the corresponding precordial
leads (V5, V6) in a child at any age. In children, T wave inversion in leads aVR and V1 is almost always normal, and T wave
inversion in lead III may also be a normal variant [5].

T wave and QRS axes are usually similar. Because of the
rightward QRS axis in the infancy period, the QRS-T angle
may be wide in this age group. The T wave axis should be in
the normal quadrant in the absence of structural heart disease
(0–90°), regardless of the QRS axis at any age. In the appropriate age group, a wide QRS-T angle may suggest myocardial dysfunction from ischemic or metabolic causes. The
differential for this finding also includes ventricular conduction disturbances or severe right or left ventricular
hypertrophy.

T wave inversions in the lateral or inferolateral leads are
abnormal in children without structural heart disease and
may suggest a cardiomyopathy. Such changes on ECG in a
child should lead to a pediatric cardiologist consult to detect
any potential pathology (Figs. 8.1 and 8.2).

T wave inversions in the precordial leads can be physio-
logic adaptation to exercise; however, this will not extend
beyond lead V4 [5, 6]. In the African American population,
these T wave inversions are also often accompanied by ST
segment changes with a particular shape and are described
below in the section on ST changes.

Q Waves: Normal or Abnormal?

The Q wave is the first initial negative deflection at the beginning of the QRS complex. A normal "benign" Q wave represents depolarization of the ventricular septum. Q waves may
be benign or pathologic. The definition of a pathologic Q
wave is a Q wave more than 5 mm deep and longer than
40 msec. The cutoff of a wide Q wave was 35 msec as stud-
ied by Towbin et al. [3], but on a 12-lead ECG, this is challenging to measure; therefore, 40 msec is a more practical
guide on a rhythm strip (one small box). Benign Q waves are
often seen in the inferior (II, III, and aVF) and lateral leads
(V4, V5, V6). Deep Q waves which are not wide may be seen
in certain congenital heart lesions, particularly those with
single-ventricle physiology, isolated ventricular hypertrophy, or cardiomyopathy.

The pathophysiologic basis of Q waves will vary depending on the disease process. Q waves in hypertrophic cardiomyopathy (HCM) are usually >3 mm deep and/or >40 ms in
duration in at least two leads [5, 7]. The Q waves of HCM are
most often seen in the inferior and/or lateral leads. Small Q
waves in these leads with no increase in width are unlikely
secondary to ischemia, infarction, or cardiomyopathy and
are more likely a result of normal septal depolarization.

Deep, narrow, Q waves (>5 mm in amplitude) are often
seen as a normal finding in younger children, infants, and
toddlers. The Q waves in these children are usually prominent in leads aVF and V6 and can be as large as 6 mm. These
Q waves are a normal variant and not synonymous with cardiac disease when noted as an isolated finding (Fig. 8.3).

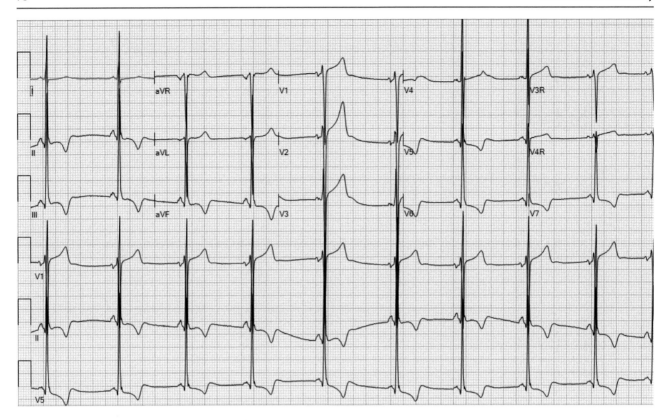

Fig. 8.1 Seventeen-year-old male with aortic stenosis, lost to follow-up. He had chest pain with exercise that led to a cardiac arrest. His ECG demonstrates left ventricular hypertrophy with strain. The T wave inversions are pathologic based on their location (lateral and inferior leads)

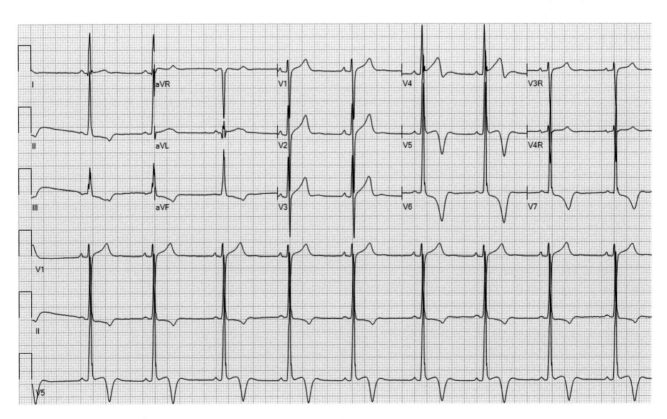

Fig. 8.2 ECG of a 15-year-old male with hypertrophic cardiomyopathy. Note the presence of inverted T waves in the inferior and lateral leads with voltage criteria for left ventricular hypertrophy

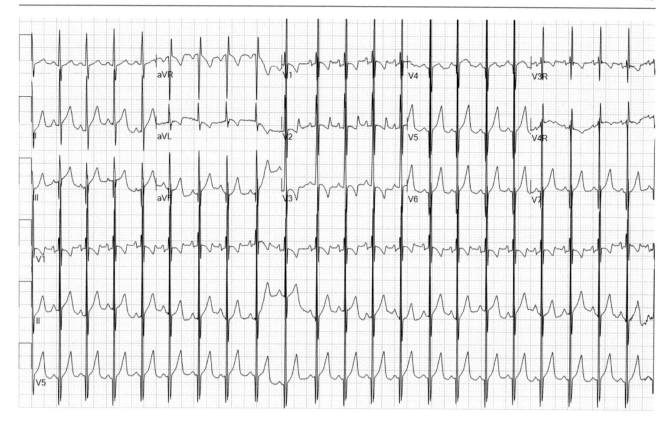

Fig. 8.3 A 9-month-old with a VSD presenting with tachypnea during feeds and poor growth prior to lasix and digoxin. Note the deep Q waves in the lateral leads (V5, V6) and inferior leads (III, aVF). The infant also meets criteria for biventricular hypertrophy. These deep Q waves can occur in scenarios of increased volume load on the ventri-cles, i.e. a VSD or PDA. The Q waves are not wide, in contrast to the Q waves seen in myocardial infarction. These non-pathologic Q waves are seen without any other abnormalities on the ECG and are considered a normal variant in toddlers

The prototype disease of pathologic Q waves in pediatric cardiology is anomalous left artery arising from the pulmonary artery (ALCAPA), previously known as Bland-Garland White syndrome. The usual presentation of this disease is an infant approximately 4–5 weeks of age who presents with symptoms of congestive heart failure. Rarely, they may present later in infancy. The classic findings on an ECG show signs of myocardial ischemia or infarction, particularly in the leads representing the left coronary artery (aVL, I, V5, V6). The ECGs of these infants are usually normal at birth because the pulmonary vascular resistance (PVR) is high, so the higher PA pressures allow for normal perfusion pressures in the anomalous coronary artery. As PVR falls in the first 3 months of life, there is reduced flow to the left coronary artery and the infant can present in extremis from cardiogenic shock. At this point in presentation, the ECG will demonstrate localized ischemic changes in the region of the left coronary artery or frank infarction (Fig. 8.4).

ST Segment Changes

The ST segment is the isoelectric segment between the QRS complex and the T wave and is the portion of the ECG where signs of ischemia and early infarction are often manifest when symptomatic patients present for evaluation (during the hyperacute phase). It represents the brief period between ventricular depolarization and repolarization. ST segments are usually flat; however there is a range of what is considered normal for the ST segment. To determine if the ST segment is flat, one has to evaluate its position in reference to the PQ and TP segments, which should also be flat. Evaluation of the ST segment requires noting the shape of the segment and the degree of change from the baseline. The change in the ST segment up to 1 mm in the limb leads is considered normal. In the precordial leads, change in the ST segment is considered normal up to 2 mm, but other features have to be considered such as the presence of T wave changes, the shape of the ST segment, and the presence of pathologic Q waves. The ST segment can have an upward sloping shape or a

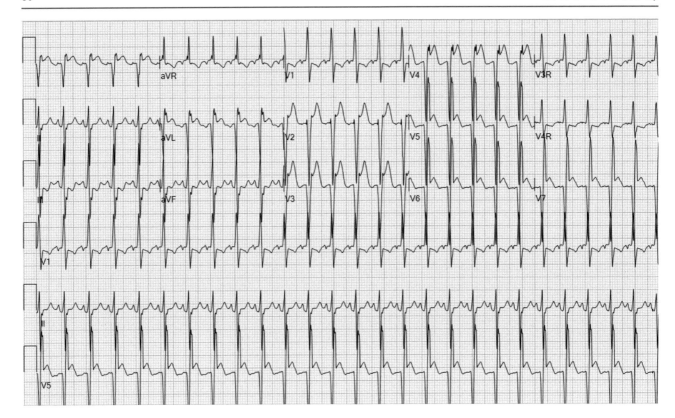

Fig. 8.4 A 4-month-old presented with cough and increased work of breathing and was found to have an enlarged cardiac silhouette on chest X-ray. After a 20 cc/kg fluid bolus, the infant's perfusion worsened and was noted to have an enlarged liver. An ECG was obtained due to cardio-megaly in the chest X-ray. The ECG revealed pathologic Q waves in I, aVL, V5, and V6 and significant ST segment elevations in the precordial leads (>2mm). The echocardiogram supported the ECG findings suggestive of ALCAPA and the patient underwent surgical repair that day

concave shape and be considered normal (assuming no other concerning findings on the ECG). Downsloping or horizontal ST segments are considered abnormal, particularly if they meet the 1 or 2 mm change in baseline criteria (depending on if they are in the limb or precordial leads). Pathologic ST segment changes are noted in a variety of conditions, such as with post-operative coronary perfusion compromise after surgical repair of d-TGA (Fig. 8.5).

The most common nonischemic cause of ST elevation in young people is early repolarization. This is a specific ST segment pattern observed frequently in adolescents, particularly athletes and African-American males. In rare cases, the degree of ST elevation can be quite profound. Early repolarization pattern on an ECG requires three criteria: (1) the presence of the J-point deviation from baseline by >0.01 mV in at least two contiguous leads, (2) the morphology of J point is described as slurred or notched, and (3) the ST segment from the J point to the T wave is described as ascending, descending (rare), or horizontal [8]. The ST segment in this context often takes a concave shape and slopes upward. The ST elevation often does not elevate >2 mm, even in athletes (Figs. 8.6 and 8.7).

In recent years the definition of early repolarization has expanded to differentiate benign vs malignant phenotypes, but this differentiation has not been validated in the pediatric population. Early repolarization has classically been described in the precordial leads but can be found in any lead. A new definition of early repolarization that is considered benign is a slur on the downslope of the R wave (Fig. 8.8) [6].

Other causes of ST elevation in children with chest pain are pericarditis and myocarditis. These are conditions defined by inflammation of the subepicardial myocardium with or without pericardial effusion. The ECG findings of acute pericarditis are well documented and can often be mistaken for early repolarization. Often the pattern of concave ST segment elevation with J-point elevation is seen more diffusely in multiple coronary artery distributions and may be observed in virtually all the leads [9] (Fig. 8.9). However, other ECG changes may be noted that are often under-recognized. The ST elevations in acute pericarditis may or may not be associated with PR segment depression, and in lead aVR there is often PR segment elevation [10]. As the disease progresses, the ST segment normalizes, and over days to weeks from initial presentation, the T waves will invert when the ST segment is isoelectric and this may persist for weeks. The ECG changes seen in acute myopericarditis evolve more gradually than the sudden ECG changes seen in a typical STEMI (ST

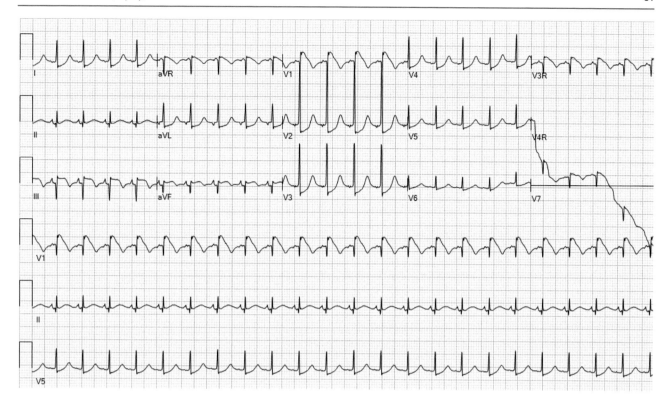

Fig. 8.5 ST elevation in an infant with myocardial infarction several hours after repair of D-transposition of the great arteries, likely related to obstruction of the right coronary artery. Note the pathologic ST seg-ment elevations in the anterior (V1) and inferior leads (III and aVF) with reciprocal pathologic ST segment depression in the mid precordial (V2–V4) and lateral leads (I and aVL)

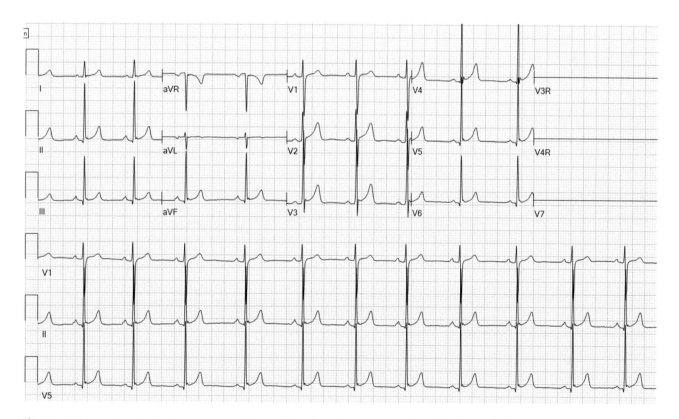

Fig. 8.6 Early repolarization in a 17-year-old male. The ST elevations have a concave shape in the lateral (V5, V6) and inferior leads (II, III, and aVF) and do not exceed 2 mm. There is a clear J wave (notched type) with J-point elevation (II, V5, and V6)

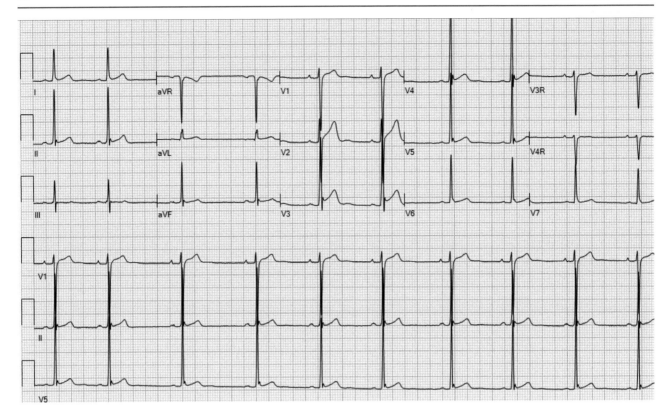

Fig. 8.7 Early repolarization in a 17-year-old male. The ST segment elevations are less than 2 mm. The terminal QRS is slurred in some leads (I, aVL, and V6) and notched in others (V4, V5)

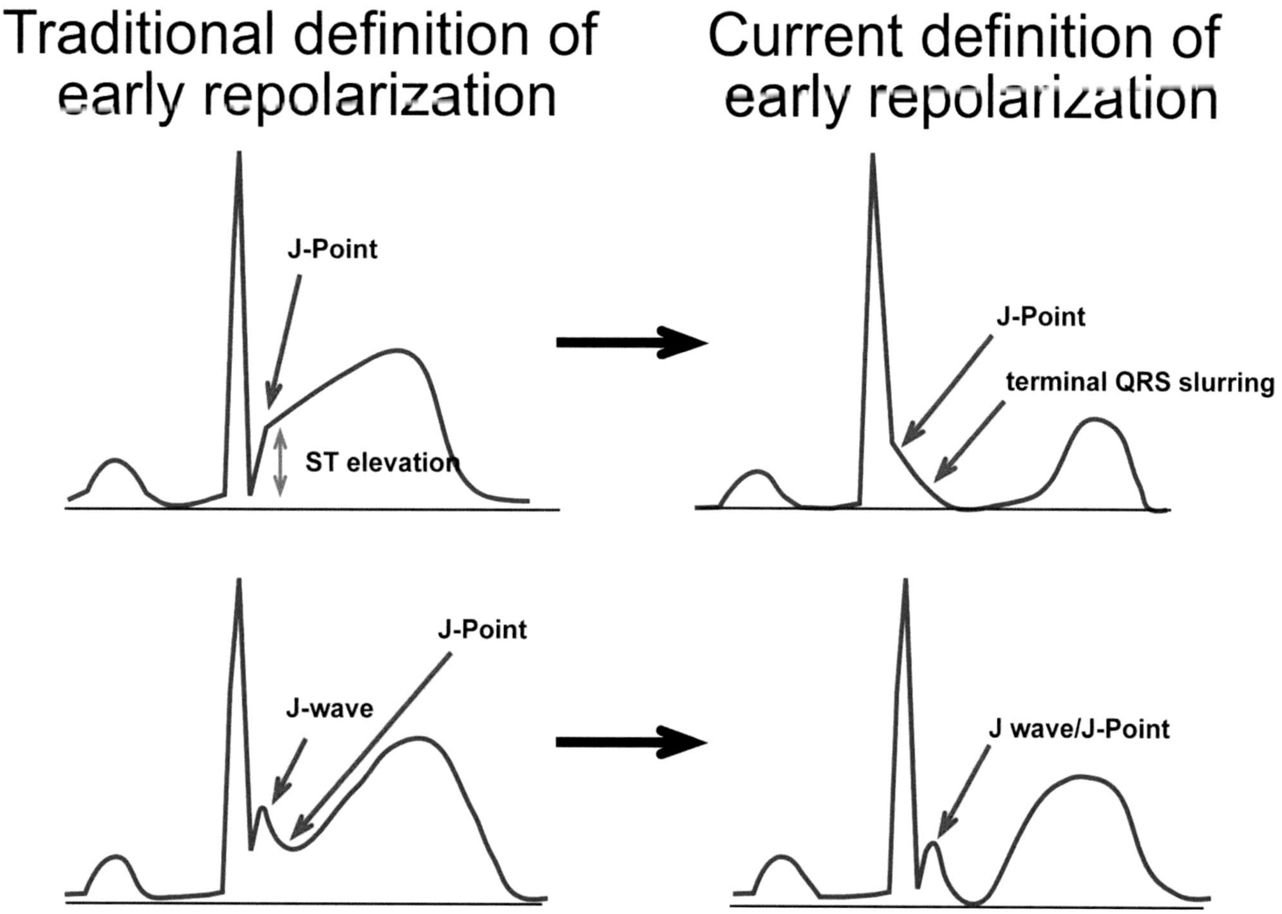

Traditional definition of early repolarization

Current definition of early repolarization

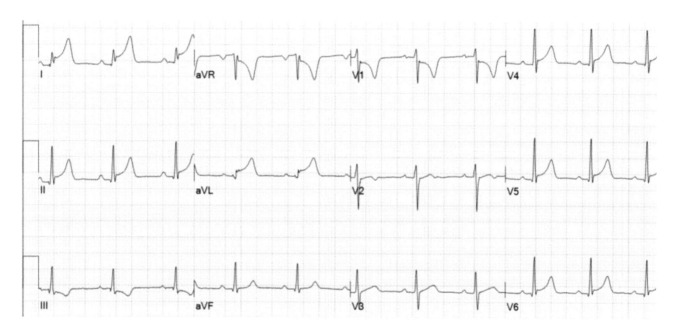

Fig. 8.8 Diagrams on the left are classic examples of early repolarization based on ST elevation at the QRS end (J-point). The bottom left diagram has a clear J wave. The diagrams on the right are examples of newer definitions of early repolarization showing a slurred QRS downstroke and J wave. The lower right diagram has no associated ST elevation

Fig. 8.9 Seventeen-year-old male with pericarditis who presented with chest pain; troponin levels were elevated. Note the ST elevations are >2 mm in leads I, II, aVL, V4, V5, and V6 and there is ST depression with T wave inversion in V1, III, and aVR

elevation myocardial infarction). This highlights the importance of serial ECGs when these patients are initially evaluated and admitted to an inpatient unit for workup and evaluation. The PR segment changes are less likely to occur in true STEMI and the leads involved in a STEMI will follow a coronary artery distribution. The presence of elevated cardiac enzymes also helps to narrow the diagnosis.

Conclusion

The ECG is a useful screening test in the evaluation of a pediatric patient with suspected myocardial ischemia or infarction. Data in the pediatric population is scarce in the absence of larger studies and criteria are mostly adapted from adult consensus statements and practice guidelines. In combination with other diagnostic modalities and good clinical judgment, the ECG can still be a useful tool to rule out acute myocardial injury but should never replace a thorough history and physical exam.

References

1. Thygesen K, Alpert JS, Jaffe AS, et al. Third universal definition of myocardial infarction. J Am Coll Cardiol. 2012;60(16):1581–98.

2. Wagner GS, Macfarlane P, Wellens H, et al. AHA/ACCF/HRS recommendations for the standardization and interpretation of the electrocardiogram: part VI: acute ischemia/infarction: a scientific statement from the American Heart Association Electrocardiography and Arrhythmias Committee, Council on Clinical Cardiology; the American College of Cardiology Foundation; and the Heart Rhythm Society: endorsed by the International Society for Computerized Electrocardiology. Circulation. 2009;119(10):e262–70.

3. Towbin JA, Bricker JT, Garson Jr A. Electrocardiographic criteria for diagnosis of acute myocardial infarction in childhood. Am J Cardiol. 1992;69(19):1545–8.

4. Gazit AZ, Avari JN, Balzer DT, Rhee EK. Electrocardiographic diagnosis of myocardial ischemia in children: is a diagnostic electrocardiogram always diagnostic? Pediatrics. 2007;120(2):440–4.

5. Drezner JA, Ashley E, Baggish AL, et al. Abnormal electrocardiographic findings in athletes: recognising changes suggestive of cardiomyopathy. Br J Sports Med. 2013;47(3):137–52.

6. Drezner JA, Fischbach P, Froelicher V, et al. Normal electrocardiographic findings: recognising physiological adaptations in athletes. Br J Sports Med. 2013;47(3):125–36.

7. Uberoi A, Stein R, Perez MV, et al. Interpretation of the electrocardiogram of young athletes. Circulation. 2011;124(6):746–57.

8. Tanguturi VK, Noseworthy PA, Newton-Cheh C, Baggish AL. The electrocardiographic early repolarization pattern in athletes: normal variant or sudden death risk factor? Sports Med (Auckland, NZ). 2012;42(5):359–66.

9. Pollak P, Brady W. Electrocardiographic patterns mimicking ST segment elevation myocardial infarction. Cardiol Clin. 2012;30(4):601–15.

10. Spodick DH. Acute pericarditis: current concepts and practice. JAMA. 2003;289(9):1150–3.

Abnormalities in Electrocardiogram Secondary to Systemic Pathology

Carlos Miranda, Brieann Muller, Anas Taqatqa, Jessie Hu, and Ra-id Abdulla

ECG Changes Secondary to Abnormal Electrolytes

Introduction

Myocardial depolarization and repolarization is the result of changes in cellular ionic permeability. The main ions involved in myocardial contractility are potassium, sodium, and calcium. While mild deviation of normal levels of these ions does not cause obvious abnormalities in myocardial function, moderate to severe changes do. Each ion is responsible for one phase or more of the action potential and its derangement will lead to certain diagnostic pattern on surface ECG. In this chapter, these diagnostic patterns are reviewed.

Potassium

Hyperkalemia

There are multiple etiologies of hyperkalemia including renal disease, congenital adrenal hyperplasia, or iatrogenic potassium overdose. As levels of serum potassium rise, pathognomonic changes can be seen on the ECG.

At serum levels of 5.5–6.5 meq/L, the T waves become taller and more peaked (Fig. 9.1). This change is due to the role of potassium in repolarization of myocytes. This however has poor positive and negative predictive value as T waves appear peaked in many normal subjects in the pediatric age groups and T wave changes are likely to be absent in children with hyperkalemia.

C. Miranda, MD • B. Muller • A. Taqatqa, MD • J. Hu, MD
R. Abdulla, MD (✉)
Pediatric Cardiology, Rush University Medical
Center, Chicago, IL, USA
e-mail: Carlos_D_Miranda@rush.edu; brieann_a_muller@rush.edu;
Anas_Taqtqa@rush.edu; Jessie_J_Hu@rush.edu;
rabdulla@rush.edu

Potassium levels over 6.6 meq/L may lead to widening of the QRS or result in bundle branch block (Fig. 9.2 a, b). This is due to a decreased potassium gradient, resulting in a resting membrane potential which is less negative, from −90 to −70 mV. Vmax of phase 0 of the action potential is greatest when the resting membrane potential is −75 mV and Vmax does not increase with a more negative resting membrane potential; therefore, the myocytes depolarize at a slower pace. This causes interventricular conduction delay, which may manifest as a specific bundle branch block, fascicular block, or diffuse QRS widening which leads to bizarre QRS complexes that may be combined with ST elevation.

Potassium level over 7.0 meq/L causes delay in conduction in the atria, manifesting as wide P wave (Fig. 9.3). Potassium levels over 8.5 meq/L causes the P wave to disappear. The SA node is relatively impervious to hyperkalemia so the SA node can directly conduct through atrial Purkinje fibers to the AV node and to the ventricles, which is called "sinoventricular conduction."

Potassium levels at around 9.0 meq/L will cause AV blocks (Fig. 9.4), ventricular tachycardia (Fig. 9.5), and ventricular fibrillation (Fig. 9.6) [1–3].

Hypokalemia

Hypokalemia is often caused by potassium loss through vomiting and diarrhea or due to iatrogenic lack of potassium intake. Other etiological factors include Cushing's disease, hyperaldosteronism, acquired renal disease, and secondary to diuretic medications.

Hypokalemia causes a lengthening of phase 3 of the action potential and a slowing of repolarization. The T-wave amplitude is decreased with occasional ST depression, and the U-wave amplitude is increased (Fig. 9.7). Hypokalemia may cause prolongation of the QTc with minimal QRS prolongation. Arrhythmias are rare unless the patient is receiving digoxin. Digoxin arrhythmogenic effects are enhanced by hypokalemia [1–3].

© Springer International Publishing Switzerland 2016
R. Abdulla et al. (eds.), *Pediatric Electrocardiography: An Algorithmic Approach to Interpretation*,
DOI 10.1007/978-3-319-26258-1_9

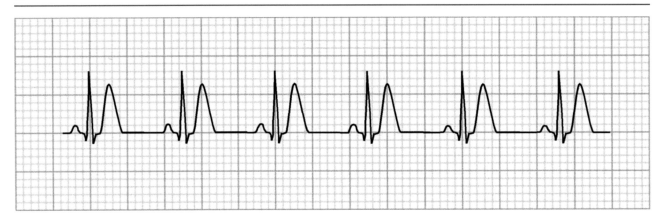

Fig. 9.1 Tall and peaked T wave in a patient with hyperkalemia

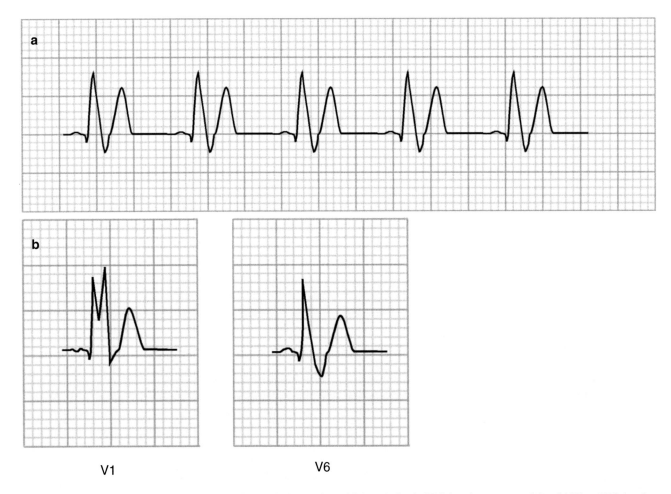

V1   V6

Fig. 9.2 (**a**) Lead II ECG demonstrating wide QRS complex in a patient with hyperkalemia QRS duration measures 1.4 s. (**b**) V1 and V6 showing right bundle branch block in a patient with hyperkalemia

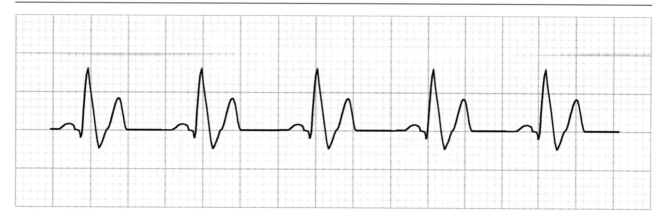

Fig. 9.3 Lead II in a patient with hyperkalemia; note the wide P wave and prolonged QRS duration

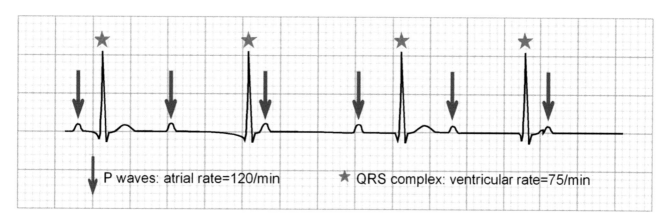

Fig. 9.4 Severe hyperkalemia in a patient with renal failure; note AV blocks (complete heart block)

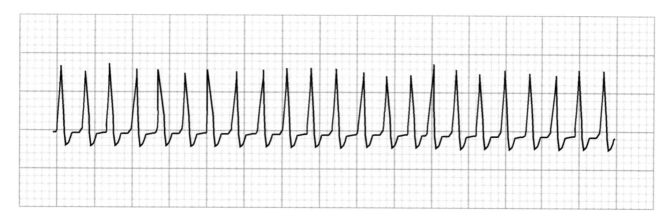

Fig. 9.5 Severe hyperkalemia in a patient with renal failure; patient presented in cardiogenic shock; note ventricular tachycardia in this lead II rhythm strip

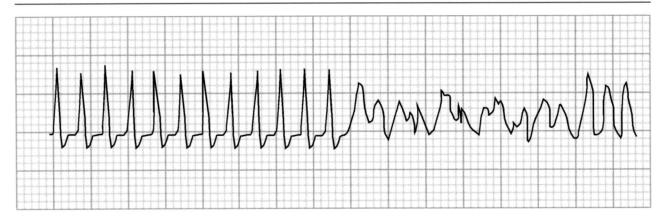

Fig. 9.6 Severe hyperkalemia in the same patient of previous figure with renal failure; ventricular fibrillation developed after a period of ventricular tachycardia

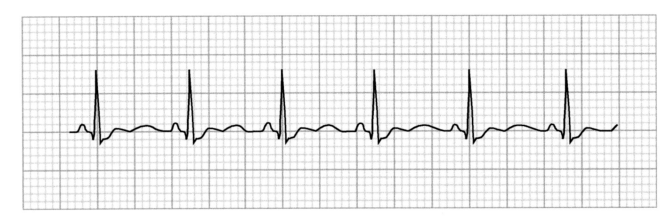

Fig. 9.7 Patient with hypokalemia demonstrating decreased T-wave amplitude with ST depression and increased U wave amplitude in lead II rhythm strip

Calcium

Hypercalcemia

Hypercalcemia can be due to hyperparathyroidism, hypophosphatasia, hypervitaminosis D, idiopathic hypercalcemia, or iatrogenic calcium infusion.

Hypercalcemia causes phase 2 of the action potential to be shortened which shortens the ST segment. Hypercalcemia affects the SA node by causing slower sinus rate, sinoatrial block, or sinus arrest. Arrhythmias are uncommon unless the patient is taking digoxin (digoxin arrhythmogenic effects are enhanced by hypercalcemia) [4–6].

Hypocalcemia

Hypocalcemia may be caused by hypoparathyroidism, vitamin D deficiency, malabsorption, or lack of calcium intake.

Hypocalcemia prolongs phase 2 of the action potential, which causes the ST segment to lengthen (Fig. 9.8). The T-wave duration is normal, but the QT interval is prolonged

because of the prolonged ST segment and late onset of the T wave. Despite prolonged QT interval, arrhythmias are rare, likely due to uniform prolongation throughout the ventricular cycle.

In newborn babies, the interval from the onset of the QRS (Q) to the onset of the T wave (OT) (Q-OT interval) correlates well with the serum calcium. The normal Q-OT in full-term newborn babies is 0.19 ms or less, and the normal Q-OT in premature infants is 0.20 ms or less. If the Q-OT is prolonged, then hypocalcemia less than 7.5 mg/dL (whole serum level) can be suspected in newborn babies [4, 5].

Magnesium

Hypermagnesemia

Hypermagnesemia is usually caused by increased intake of magnesium but may be seen in renal failure as well.

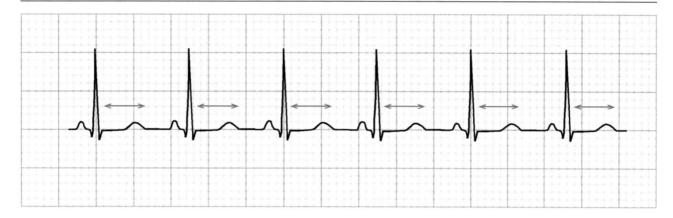

Fig. 9.8 Lead II rhythm strip in a patient with hypocalcemia. The T-wave duration is normal, but the QT interval is prolonged because of the prolonged ST segment and late onset of the T wave. *Blue arrow* indicates ST segment

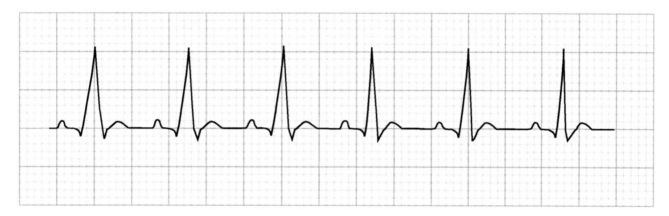

Fig. 9.9 Prolonged PR interval, increased QRS duration, and ST segment shortening in a lead II rhythm strip in a patient with hypermagnesemia

Hypermagnesemia simulates hypercalcemia, where phase 2 of the action potential is shortened. Hypermagnesemia alone produces few changes on ECG until magnesium level reaches 6–12 mg/dL. These changes include prolonged PR interval, increased QRS duration, and ST segment shortening (Fig. 9.9) and therefore shorter QTc [4, 5].

Hypomagnesemia
Hypomagnesemia is caused by GI or renal losses. GI losses include acute or chronic diarrhea, malabsorption, steatorrhea, and small bowel bypass surgery. Renal losses can occur due to organic causes such as familial renal magnesium wasting, primary aldosteronism, and uncontrolled diabetes mellitus. It may also occur due to acquired causes such as acute kidney injury, diuretics, nephrotoxins, and chronic alcohol use.

The effects of hypomagnesemia are similar to those of combined hypocalcemia and hypokalemia. The action potential has a prolonged plateau and slower descent. ECG changes include large U waves with flattened T waves and long ST segment and therefore prolonged QTc [4, 5].

Sodium

Increased sodium concentration causes an increase in the slope of phase 0 and prolonged phase 3. However at levels physiologically possible in the body, sodium does not cause changes visible on ECG [4, 5].

Hypoxia/Acidosis

Acidosis causes ECG changes similar to those of hyperkalemia, although this may be due to hydrogen ion exchange into the cell and potassium ions out of the cell. Prolonged QRS and prolonged QT are seen (Fig. 9.10) and can progress to atrial and ventricular arrhythmias as well as AV block [4, 5].

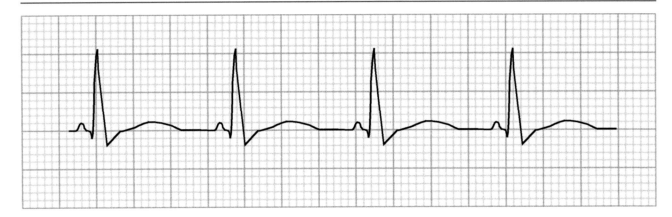

Fig. 9.10 Prolonged QRS and QT duration in a patient with severe acidosis

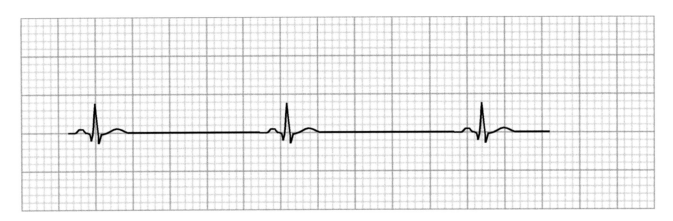

Fig. 9.11 Rhythm strip, lead II in a patient with hypothyroidism showing sinus bradycardia and low-voltage QRS complex

ECG Changes Secondary to Systemic Disease

Introduction

Cardiac involvement with systemic pathology can be differentiated broadly into two categories. Cardiac manifestations may occur as a result of systemic disease or as part of a syndrome with a collection of systemic findings, usually as part of a genetic syndrome. This section will focus on the former and discuss the various systemic diseases which affect the heart and are manifest on ECG.

Hypothyroidism

Mechanism If congenital, symptoms subtly progress in the first weeks to months of life. Symptoms can include bradycardia, low pulse pressure, heart murmur, and pericardial effusion [7–9].

ECG Findings/Rhythm Disturbances Sinus bradycardia; QRS complex may have low voltage; and shortened QTc [3] (Fig. 9.11).

Hyperthyroidism

Mechanism In the congenital variant, most newborns are symptomatic at birth with tachycardia, tachypnea, elevated temperature, palpitations, and elevated systemic pressures [7].

ECG Findings/Rhythm Disturbances Sinus tachycardia and nonspecific ST segment, and T-wave changes may be seen. Atrial fibrillation may sometimes be seen as the initial presentation [8] (Fig. 9.12).

Cushing Syndrome (Excess Cortisol)

Mechanism Cardiovascular consequence is secondary to elevation of cortisol or other glucocorticoids [7]. Hypertension may lead to LV hypertrophy over time and eventually to heart failure.

ECG Findings/Rhythm Disturbances Increased left ventricular voltage (Fig. 9.13).

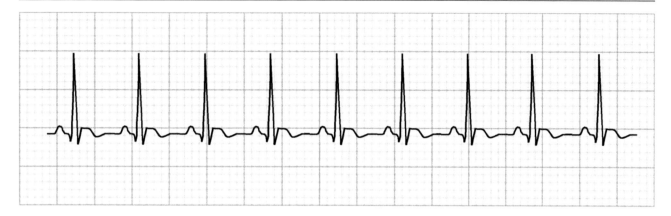

Fig. 9.12 Rhythm strip, lead II in a patient with hyperthyroidism showing sinus tachycardia and nonspecific ST segment changes

Fig. 9.13 LVH in a patient with Cushing's syndrome

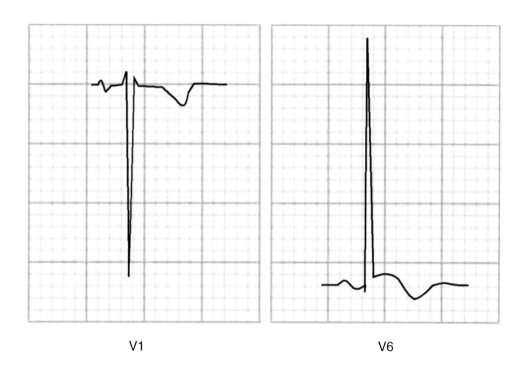

V1   V6

Adrenocortical Insufficiency (Addison Disease)

Mechanism Acquired primary adrenocortical insufficiency is termed Addison disease. Addison disease is caused by auto-immune destruction of the adrenal glands results in hypotension and decreased cardiac output. Electrolyte imbalances include hyponatremia and hyperkalemia [7]. ECG can be useful for quickly detecting hyperkalemia in a critically ill child.

ECG Findings/Rhythm Disturbances Depending on the potassium level, hyperkalemia will generally produce tall peaked T, QRS widening, and PR prolongation. This can later lead to ventricular fibrillation at potassium levels above 9 mEq/L [12] (Figs. 9.2, 9.3, 9.4, 9.5, and 9.6).

Infectious Diseases

HIV

Cardiac Involvement The cardiovascular consequences may be secondary to HIV, opportunistic infections, and side effects of medications. Before medications were introduced, there was a 4–28 % incidence of heart failure. Atherosclerosis, dilated cardiomyopathy, left ventricular dysfunction, pulmonary hypertension, infective endocarditis, malignancies, and vasculitis are some of the HIV-associated cardiovascular diseases mentioned [10].

ECG Findings/Rhythm Disturbances Will depend largely on the specific cardiac involvement. Right ventricular

Fig. 9.14 A patient with HIV showing RVH, ST, and T changes and prolonged QTc

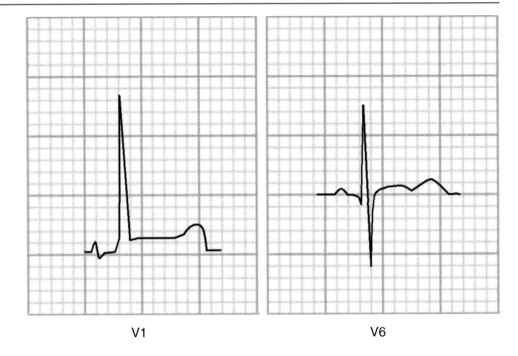

V1   V6

hypertrophy due to pulmonary hypertension secondary to multiple pulmonary viral infections, low-voltage QRS complex secondary to heart failure, nonspecific ST segment and T-wave changes possibly secondary to coronary artery disease, and prolonged QTc interval leading possibly to sudden death especially in HIV patients with hepatitis C coinfection [10] (Fig. 9.14).

Lyme Disease

Cardiac Involvement The incidence of cardiac involvement has been previously reported in about 8 % of those exposed. In those with Lyme carditis, atrioventricular node block is the most common cardiac manifestation but usually self-limiting. Other rare findings have been dilated cardiomyopathy and myopericarditis [11, 12].

ECG Findings/Rhythm Disturbances ST and T changes reflecting myocarditis and varying degrees of AV block [12] (Figs. 9.15 and 9.16).

Chagas' Disease

Cardiac Involvement Through the disease process complex pathogenesis, there are both acute and chronic cardiac manifestations. Acute myocarditis may lead to heart failure and possibly death, while the chronic Chagas' disease may present with dilated cardiomyopathy. Other manifestations such as heart block and tachyarrhythmia may become evident and an indication of a worse prognosis [13].

ECG Findings/Rhythm Disturbances Low-voltage QRS complexes with tachycardia can be seen in those with myocarditis along with prolonged P-R interval, arrhythmias, and heart block [13] (Fig. 9.17).

Trichinosis

Cardiac Involvement Trichinosis may cause myocarditis or myopericarditis [14].

ECG Findings/Rhythm Disturbances Nonspecific ST-T wave changes, bundle branch block (RBBB), supraventricular and ventricular extra systoles, and sinus tachycardia [14].

Diphtheria

Cardiac Involvement Acute inflammation can occur likely secondary to the direct action of the diphtheria toxin, leading to myocarditis. ECG changes may be a reflection of the myocardial involvement and, to a lesser extent AV conduction abnormalities. In a study be Lumio et al., of 122 patients with diphtheria, 28 % had ECG changes with a median time from symptom onset to an abnormal ECG of about 9 days [15].

ECG Findings/Rhythm Disturbances ST changes, T wave inversion, and QTc prolongation were among the most common ECG findings. Conduction abnormalities were also appreciated [15].

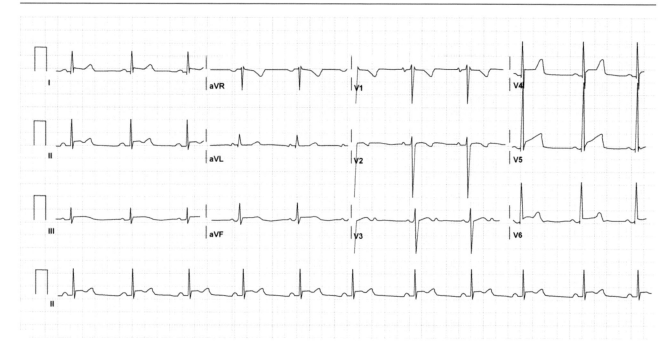

Fig. 9.15 12-lead ECG in a patient with myopericarditis secondary to Lyme disease: ST segment elevations in the inferior and precordial leads

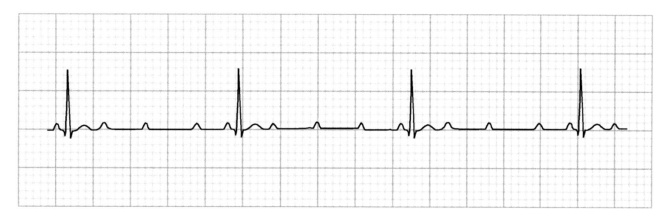

Fig. 9.16 Patient with Lyme disease and second-degree heart block

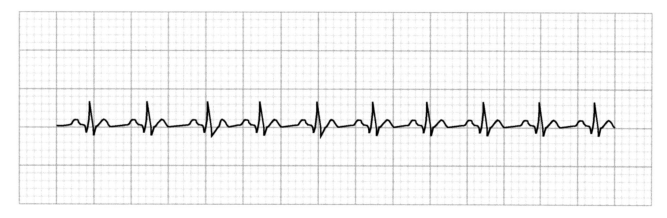

Fig. 9.17 A patient with Chagas' disease manifesting with low-voltage QRS complexes with tachycardia

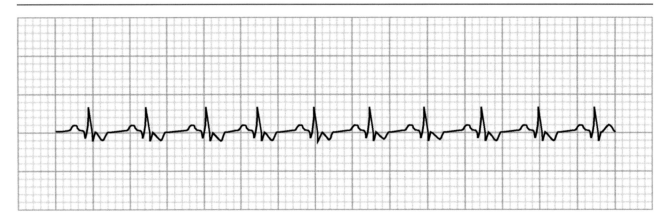

Fig. 9.18 A patient with myocarditis. ECG shows sinus tachycardia with low-voltage QRS complexes and T-wave inversion

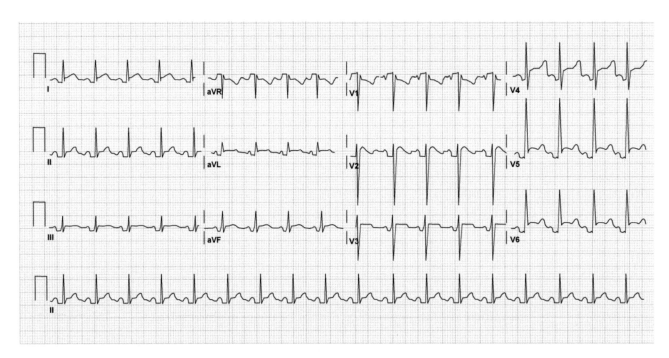

Fig. 9.19 Patient with pericarditis: PR segment is depressed while ST is elevated in I, II, III, aVL, aVF, and V2-6. Reciprocal changes in leads aVR and V1. Sinus tachycardia may reflect pericardial effusion

Myocarditis, Pericarditis

Myocarditis
Cardiac Involvement Myocarditis is the cause of dilated cardiomyopathy in children in about 46 % of the cases [16]. Of those diagnosed with myocarditis, viral infection has been the most likely cause, but other nonviral causes, whether infectious, toxic, autoimmune, or drug associated, have been well described [8, 17].

ECG Findings/Rhythm Disturbances The most common features include sinus tachycardia in possible combination with low-voltage QRS complexes along with T-wave inversion [8] (Fig. 9.18).

Pericarditis

Cardiac Involvement Primary involvement of the pericardium is likely rare, but involvement secondary to systemic disease such as autoimmune disorders, renal diseases, mediastinal lymph node enlargement (lymphoma, granulomatous disease), mediastinal teratoma, and traumatic consequences have all been well described [8].

ECG Findings/Rhythm Disturbances Early ECG finding may include early PR-segment abnormalities before classic findings, which include diffuse ST elevation and PR depression [18, 19] (Fig. 9.19).

Neurological Disorders

Muscular Dystrophies: Duchenne and Becker

Cardiac Involvement The majority develops cardiomyopathy over time, which may sometimes be masked by skeletal muscle weakness [20]. Nigro et al. showed that preclinical cardiac involvement was found in 25 % of patients less than 6 years of age, while clinical evidence of cardiomyopathy is initially seen after 10 years of age [21].

ECG Findings Sinus tachycardia, tall R waves, and increased R/S amplitude in V1 and deep narrow Q waves in the left precordial leads related to ventricular involvement [22].

Myotonic Dystrophy

Cardiac Involvement Myotonic dystrophy is primary muscular disorder that has been shown to cause sudden death in roughly one third of patients who have died from a cardiac cause [23, 24]. When there is cardiac involvement, it is primarily affecting the conduction system from the sinus node to the His-Purkinje fibers leading to an age-dependent risk of arrhythmias [25, 26].

ECG Findings Variable conduction abnormalities can be observed. Independent risk factors for sudden death can include a PR interval >240 ms, a QRS duration > 120 ms, or evidence of second- or third-degree AV block [27].

Friedreich's Ataxia

Cardiac Involvement Neurologic symptoms typically manifest at puberty and almost always before 25 years of age. Most neurologically symptomatic patients have cardiac abnormalities, primarily findings of ventricular hypertrophy. Approximately 70 % of patients will have an abnormal echocardiogram, with the majority showing increased wall thickness and, more rarely, systolic dysfunction [28–30].

ECG Findings Atrial arrhythmias, including flutter and fibrillation, can be associated with progression to a dilated cardiomyopathy. Ventricular tachycardia in the setting of dilated cardiomyopathy has been observed. Sudden death can occur with a mechanism that has not been well characterized [31].

Increased Intracranial Pressure (ICP)

Cardiac Involvement ECG changes depends upon etiology of ICP. An increase in sympathetic and vagal activity may be seen in patients with subarachnoid hemorrhage [32]. Tumors may lead to a mass effect of the limbic structures, which could exert arrhythmogenic effects [33].

ECG Findings It is possible to appreciate tall P waves, prolongation of the QTc, and extrasystoles from a sympathetic consequence of ICP. Prominent U waves are specific to intracranial hemorrhage. Other notable changes can include sinus bradycardia and ST and T-wave changes [34, 35].

Connective Tissue Disease

Systemic Lupus Erythematosus (SLE)

Cardiac Involvement SLE is a rheumatic disease seen in both adults and children. Cardiac involvement is common and may include all layers of the heart, noninfectious endocarditis, and thrombosis. Occasionally older children may develop conduction and rhythm abnormalities [36].

ECG Changes AV block, intraventricular conduction problems, and sick sinus syndrome have been appreciated along with sinus tachycardia, atrial fibrillation, atrial ectopy, and long QT syndrome [36, 37].

ECG Changes Secondary to Pharmacological Agents

Many medications interfere with the normal electrophysiology of the heart and can cause electrocardiogram (ECG) changes, even at nontoxic levels. Some of these changes are benign and well tolerated, while others may lead to deleterious effects and are indications to discontinue the agent. It is essential to have basic knowledge of cardiac physiology, in order to understand the ECG changes associated with various pharmacologic agents.

The main mechanisms of these agents include membrane-depressant action as in sodium channel blockers, calcium channel blockers, outward potassium (K+) channel blockers, and sodium-potassium adenosine-triphosphatase blockers, as well as alterations of the autonomic nervous system and its sites of cardiovascular action as in beta-adrenergic blockers and other sympathetic inhibitors and sympathomimetic, anticholinergic, and cholinomimetic substances.

In this section, some of the more commonly used drug categories leading to ECG changes are discussed [38–40].

Anti-arrhythmic

Digoxin
   ECG changes include:

- Sinus bradycardia
- Prolonged PR

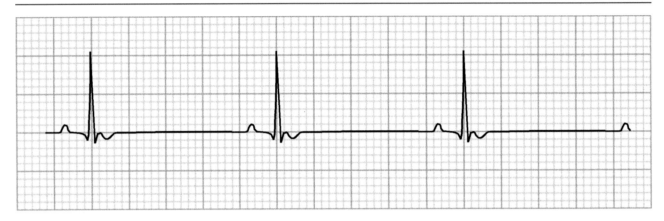

Fig. 9.20 Rhythm strip of a patient using digoxin; note sinus bradycardia, prolonged PR interval, shortened QT interval, and T-wave inversion

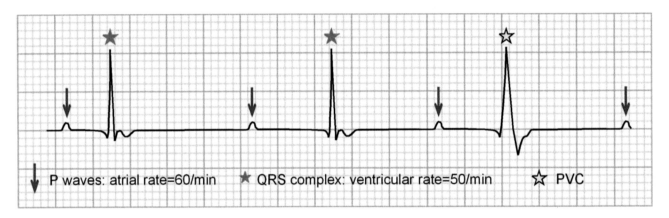

↓ P waves: atrial rate=60/min   ★ QRS complex: ventricular rate=50/min   ☆ PVC

Fig. 9.21 A 2-year-old child who accidentally ingested grandmother's digoxin pills. Digoxin serum level was 3.2 ng/ml. Rhythm strip shows sinus bradycardia, third-degree AV block, and PVCs

- Shortened QT
- ST and T wave changes
- AV block
- Toxicity: sinus arrest, second-degree AV block (type I), third-degree AV block, and ventricular tachycardia

Digoxin has several effects on cardiac conduction. Specifically, digoxin slows the sinus node rate, decreases atrial automaticity, increases intra-atrial conduction, and prolongs AV conduction. These effects are usually manifested as sinus bradycardia and a prolonged PR interval. At the cellular level, digoxin shortens phase 2 of the action potential and shortens the entire action potential duration. With digoxin, all layers of the ventricle tend to repolarize simultaneously, resulting in greater cancellation of repolarization vector and flat T waves. The onset of repolarization is also affected which results in depressed ST segments (especially in leads facing the left ventricle). The latter portion of repolarization is unaffected so the terminal T waves appear normal. Higher doses of digoxin causes the process of repolarization to reverse (from the endocardium to the epicardium), thus resulting in T-wave inversion (Fig. 9.20).

Digoxin toxicity causes further slowing of sinus rate, resulting in atrial block and second-degree AV block (usually type 1) or third-degree AV block. If AV block and PVCs occur on same ECG, one should suspect digoxin toxicity (Fig. 9.21).

A unique observation in patients with digoxin toxicity and hypokalemia is "bidirectional **tachycardia**" where there is *constant complete right bundle branch block with alternating right and left axis deviation* (Fig. 9.22).

Quinidine/procainamide (class IA):

- Prolonged QT
- Prolonged QRS
- T wave changes
- Toxicity: sinus bradycardia, AV block, prolonged QRS (more than 125 % original QRS), premature ventricular contractions, ventricular tachycardia (torsades de pointes)

Class IA anti-arrhythmics block sodium and potassium channels which results in decreased upstroke velocity of the action potential, prolonged phase 3 (lengthened action potential duration), and reduced automaticity (Fig. 9.23). This is reflected on the ECG as interventricular conduction delay,

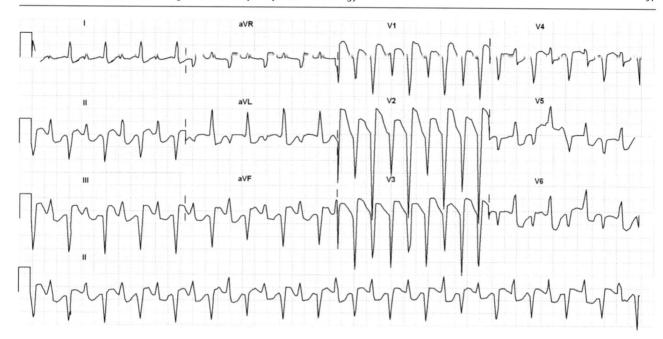

Fig. 9.22 Wide complex tachycardia (HR 320 bpm) with no appreciable P waves. QRS axis varies beat to beat from −60° to 70°

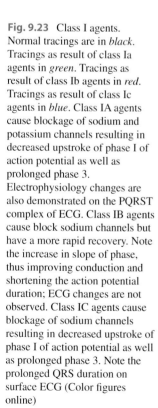

Fig. 9.23 Class I agents. Normal tracings are in *black*. Tracings as result of class Ia agents in *green*. Tracings as result of class Ib agents in *red*. Tracings as result of class Ic agents in *blue*. Class IA agents cause blockage of sodium and potassium channels resulting in decreased upstroke of phase I of action potential as well as prolonged phase 3. Electrophysiology changes are also demonstrated on the PQRST complex of ECG. Class IB agents cause block sodium channels but have a more rapid recovery. Note the increase in slope of phase, thus improving conduction and shortening the action potential duration; ECG changes are not observed. Class IC agents cause blockage of sodium channels resulting in decreased upstroke of phase I of action potential as well as prolonged phase 3. Note the prolonged QRS duration on surface ECG (Color figures online)

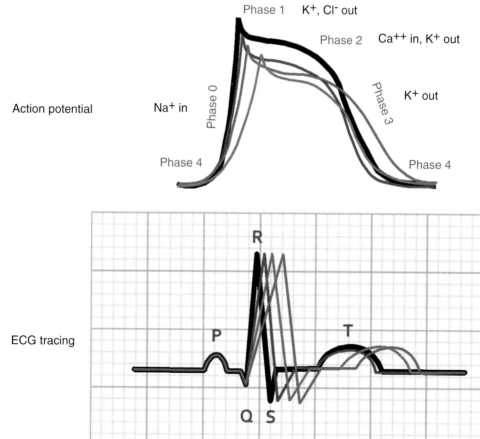

Fig. 9.24 Class II agents result in action potential and PQRST (*ECG*) changes due to reduction in upstroke of action potential results in sinus bradycardia and shortened QT interval

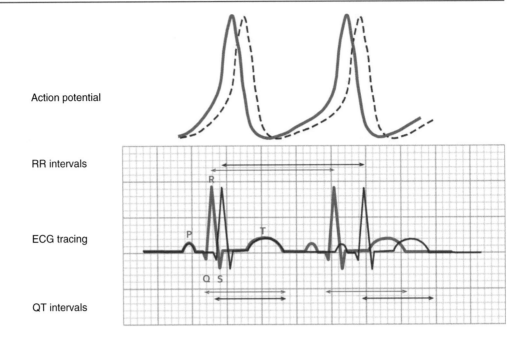

Action potential

RR intervals

ECG tracing

QT intervals

prolonged QRS duration, and prolonged QT. The QRS may be diffusely widened or more specific to the right or left bundle branch. Recovery from block is termed "intermediate" for this class specifically, which results in slightly prolonged QRS at normal heart rates and more noticeable prolongation at faster rates. Regarding T waves, terminal repolarization is most affected by these agents; this may look similar to a u wave (early T wave with low amplitude compared to late portion). PR interval may be shortened due to vagolytic effects.

Lidocaine/phenytoin/mexiletine (class IB):

• Shortened QT

Class IB agents also block sodium channels but have a more rapid recovery than class IA agents. These anti-arrhythmics increase the slope of phase 0 in diseased tissue specifically (which improves conduction) and shorten the action potential duration but have little effect on surface ECG. At rapid heart rates, the QRS prolongation is more evident. With higher doses, the PR and QT intervals may shorten due to accelerated AV conduction and shortened ventricular refractoriness. These agents tend to affect ventricular tissue more than atrial tissue (Fig. 9.23).

Flecainide/propafenone (class IC):

• Prolonged QRS

Similar to class IA and IB, class IC agents also block sodium channels but show slower recovery of channel block-ade. This results in notable QRS prolongation even at normal heart rates (Fig. 9.23).

Beta-blocking agents (class II):

• Shortened QT
• Sinus bradycardia
• Prolonged PR interval
• AV block

Beta-blockers exert their effect on cardiac cells through its anti-adrenergic effects. It causes decreased upstroke velocity of phase 0, shortened action potential duration, and decreased automaticity of cardiac cells (Fig. 9.24). These effects are mainly anti-adrenergic in etiology. Ultimately, the sinus rate is slowed, PR interval prolonged, and the QT interval may shorten.

Amiodarone/sotalol (class III):

• Prolonged QT interval

Class III agents block potassium channels which results in delayed repolarization and prolonged refractoriness. This manifests as prolonged QT and slowed AV nodal conduction (Fig. 9.25).

Verapamil/diltiazem (class IV):

• Sinus bradycardia
• AV block

These agents act as calcium antagonists with primary effects on the sinus and AV nodes. At the cellular level, class IV agents cause decreased slope of phase 0, prolonged action potential duration, and reduced automaticity. These effects are manifested as a slowed sinus rate and prolonged PR interval on ECG (Fig. 9.26).

Fig. 9.25 Class III block potassium channels resulting in delayed repolarization during phase 3, thus prolonging refractoriness. This manifests as prolonged PR and QT intervals on surface ECG

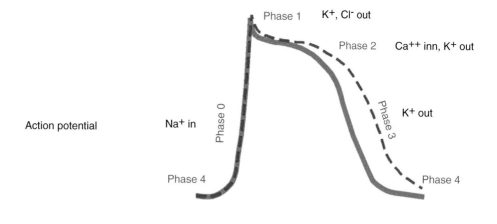

Action potential

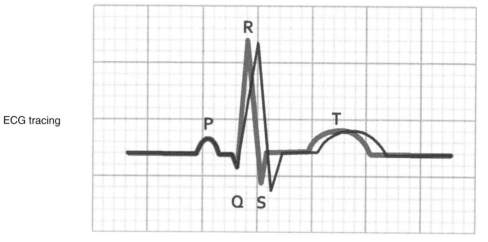

ECG tracing

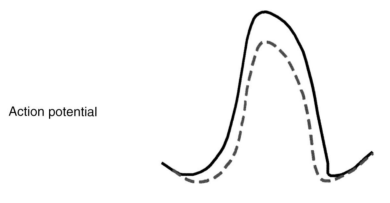

Action potential

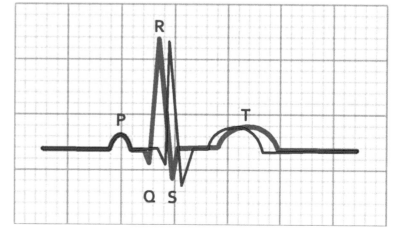

ECG tracing

Fig. 9.26 Class IV agents cause decreased slope of phase 0, prolonged action potential duration, and reduced automaticity. These effects are manifested as a slowed sinus rate and prolonged PR interval on ECG

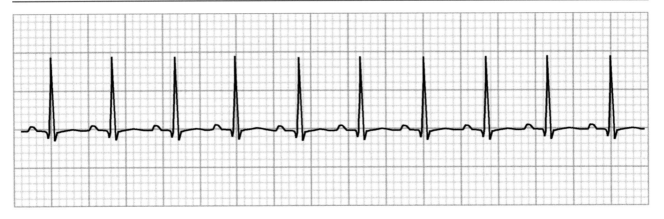

Fig. 9.27 ECG rhythm strip in a patient receiving tricyclic antidepressants. Note sinus tachycardia, prolonged PR interval, and flattened T waves

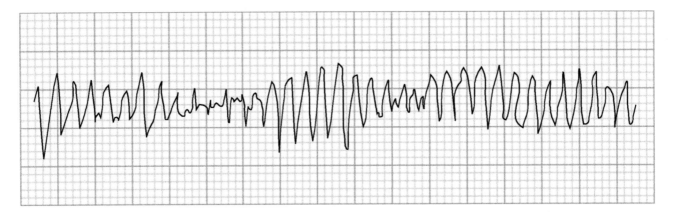

Fig. 9.28 Torsades de pointes

Anesthetic Agents

Halothane:

- Shortened QT
- Sinus bradycardia
- Toxicity: ventricular tachycardia

Halothane decreases the action potential duration by increasing the slope of phase 2 and 3. ECG changes are rare; however one may see a shortened QT interval and decreased T-wave amplitude. Because halothane sensitizes the heart to vagal and sympathetic stimulation, sinus bradycardia and ventricular arrhythmias may be seen.

Psychotropic

Tricyclic antidepressants:

- AV block
- Toxicity: atrial and ventricular arrhythmias

The mechanism behind altered cardiac conduction with these medications is related to shifts in extracellular potassium. ECG changes are observed in approximately 20 % of patients taking these medications. Specifically, sinus tachycardia, prolonged PR interval, and flat T waves are most commonly seen. QRS and QT prolongation and ST changes have been documented. Overdose with these medications may result in atrial or ventricular arrhythmias or AV block (Fig. 9.27).

Selective serotonin reuptake inhibitors (SSRIs):

- Prolonged QT interval
- Sinus bradycardia

Prolonged QT interval and sinus bradycardia may be observed. Animal models have shown inhibition of sodium and calcium channels by SSRIs.

Antipsychotics:

- Prolonged QT interval
- Ventricular tachycardia (torsades de pointes)

These medications mostly inhibit potassium channels which can lead to prolongation of the QT interval and ultimately torsades de pointes (Fig. 9.28).

Chemotherapy

Anthracyclines (daunorubicin):

- ST changes
- Premature atrial and ventricular contractions

The cardiac effects related to these chemotherapy agents are likely related to oxidative damage. Although there can be significant long-term sequelae from these medications, the ECG findings are usually transient and asymptomatic.

References

1. Pepin J, Shields C. Advances in diagnosis and management of hypokalemic and hyperkalemic emergencies. Emerg Med Pract. 2012;14(2):1–17; quiz 17–8.
2. Mandal AK. Hypokalemia and hyperkalemia. Med Clin North Am. 1997;81(3):611–39.
3. Parham WA, Mehdirad AA, Biermann KM, Fredman CS. Hyperkalemia revisited. Tex Heart Inst J. 2006;33(1):40–7.
4. Diercks DB, Shumaik GM, Harrigan RA, Brady WJ, Chan TC. Electrocardiographic manifestations: electrolyte abnormalities. J Emerg Med. 2004;27(2):153–60.
5. El-Sherif N, Turitto G. Electrolyte disorders and arrhythmogenesis. Cardiol J. 2011;18(3):233–45.
6. Gardner JD, Calkins JB, Garrison GE. ECG diagnosis: the effect of ionized serum calcium levels on electrocardiogram. Perm J. 2014;18(1):e119–20.
7. Marcdante, Karen;Kliegman, Robert M, Jenson Hal B, Behrman Richard E. (2010-03-31). Nelson essentials of pediatrics (essentials of pediatrics (Nelson)) (Kindle Locations 32364–32366). Elsevier Health. Kindle Edition, 2010.
8. Allen Hugh D, Driscoll David J, Shaddy Robert E, Feltes Timothy F. Moss & Adams' heart disease in infants, children, and adolescents: including the fetus and young adult. Lippincott Williams and Wilkins 2011.
9. Asami T, Suzuki H, Yazaki S, et al. Effects of thyroid hormone deficiency on electrocardiogram findings of congenitally hypothyroid neonates. Thyroid. 2001;11:765–8.
10. Lipshultz SE, Miller TL, Wilkinson JD, et al. Cardiac effects in perinatally HIV-infected and HIV-exposed but uninfected children and adolescents: a view from the United States of America. J Int AIDS Soc. 2013;16:18597.
11. Horowitz HW, Belkin RN. Acute myopericarditis resulting from Lyme disease. Am Heart J. 1995;130:176–8.
12. Krause P, Bockenstedt L. Lyme disease and the heart. Circulation. 2013;127:e451–4. CirculationAHA.112.101485.
13. Tanowitz H, Kirchhoff L, Simon D, et al. Chagas' disease. Clin Microbiol Rev. 1992;5:400–19.
14. Puljiz I, Beus A, Kuzman I, Seiwerth S. Electrocardiographic changes and myocarditis in trichinellosis: a retrospective study of 154 patients. Ann Trop Med Parasitol. 2005;99:403–11.
15. Lumio JT, Groundstroem KW, Melnick OB, et al. Electrocardiographic abnormalities in patients with diphtheria: a prospective study. Am J Med. 2004;116:78–83.
16. Towbin JA, et al. Incidence, causes, and outcomes of dilated cardiomyopathy in children. JAMA. 2006;296:1867–76. Allen Hugh D, Driscoll David J, Shaddy Robert E, Feltes Timothy F. (2012-11-19).
17. Berkovich S, Rodriguez-Torres R, Lin JS. Virologic studies in children with acute myocarditis. Am J Dis Child. 1968;115: 207–12. Allen Hugh D, Driscoll David J, Shaddy Robert E, Feltes Timothy F. (2012-11-19).
18. Baljepally R, Spodick DH. PR-segment deviation as initial electrocardiographic response in acute pericarditis. Am J Cardiol. 1998;81:1505–6.
19. Nalmas S, Nagarakanti R, Slim J, Abter E. Electrocardiographic changes in infectious diseases. Hosp Physician. 2007;43:15–27.
20. Romfh A, McNally EM. Cardiac assessment in Duchenne and Becker muscular dystrophies. Curr Heart Fail Rep. 2010;7:212–8.
21. Nigro G, Li C, Politano L, Bain RJ. The incidence and evolution of cardiomyopathy in Duchenne muscular dystrophy. Int J Cardiol. 1990;26:271–7.
22. Perloff JK, Roberts WC, de leon AC, O'Doherty D. The distinctive electrocardiogram of Duchenne's progressive muscular dystrophy. An electrocardiographic pathologic correlative study. Am J Med. 1967;42:179–88.
23. Mathieu J, Allard P, Potvin L, Prevost C, Begin P. A 10 year study of mortality in a cohort of patients with myotonic dystrophy. Neurology. 1999;52:1658–62.
24. de Die-Smulders CE, Höweler CJ, Thijs C, et al. Age and causes of death in adult-onset myotonic dystrophy. Brain. 1998;121(Pt 8): 1557–63.
25. Nguyen HH, Wolfe 3d JT, Holmes Jr DR, Edwards WD. Pathology of the cardiac conduction system in myotonic dystrophy: a study of 12 cases. J Am Coll Cardiol. 1988;11:662–71.
26. Lazarus A, Varin J, Babuty D, Anselme F, Coste J, Duboc D, et al. Long-term follow-up of arrhythmias in patients with myotonic dystrophy treated by pacing: a multicenter diagnostic pacemaker study. J Am Coll Cardiol. 2002;40(9). 1645Á52.
27. Groh WJ, Groh MR, Chandan S, et al. Electrocardiographic abnormalities and risk of sudden death in myotonic dystrophy type 1. N Engl J Med. 2008;358:2688–97.
28. Schulz JB, Boesch S, Burk K, Durr A, Giunti P, Mariotti C, Pousset F, Schols L, Vankan P, Pandolfo M. Diagnosis and treatment of Friedreich ataxia: a European perspective. Nat Rev Neurol. 2009; 5:222–34.
29. Durr A, Cossee M, Agid Y, Campuzano V, Mignard C, Penet C, Mandel JL, Brice A, Koenig M. Clinical and genetic abnormalities in patients with Friedreich's ataxia. N Engl J Med. 1996;335:1169–75.
30. Mottram PM, Delatycki MB, Donelan L, Gelman JS, Corben L, Peverill RE. Early changes in left ventricular long-axis function in Friedreich ataxia: relation with the FXN gene mutation and cardiac structural change. J Am Soc Echocardiogr. 2011;24:782–9.
31. Weidemann F, Rummey C, Bijnens B, et al. The heart in Friedreich ataxia: definition of cardiomyopathy, disease severity, and correlation with neurologic symptoms. Circulation. 2012;125:1626–34.
32. Kawahara E, Ikeda S, Miyahara Y, Kohno S. Role of au- role of autonomic nervous dysfunction in electrocardiographic abnormalities and cardiac injury in patients with acute subarachnoid hemorrhage. Circ J. 2003;67:753–6.
33. Koepp M, Kern A, Schmidt D. Electrocardiographic changes in patients with brain tumors. Arch Neurol. 1995;52:152–5.
34. Syverud G. Electrocardiographic changes and intracranial pathology. AANA J. 1991;59:229–32.
35. Hersch C. Electrocardiographic changes in subarachnoid haemorrhage, meningitis, and intracranial space occupying lesions. Br Heart J. 1964;26:785–93.
36. Liautaud S, et al. Variable atrioventricular block in systemic lupus erythematosus. Clin Rheumatol. 2005;24:162–5.
37. Teixeira RA, et al. Arrhythmias in systemic lupus erythematosus. Rev Bras Reumatol. 2010;50:81–9.
38. Catalina Lionte, Cristina Bologa, Laurentiu Sorodoc. Toxic and drug-induced changes of the Electrocardiogram. In: Richard M. Millis, editors. Advances in Electrocardiograms – clinical applications. InTech; 2012. p. 271–96.
39. Garson A. The electrocardiogram in infants and children: a systematic approach. Philadelphia: Lea & Febiger; 1983.
40. Wecker L, Crespo LM, Dunaway G, Faingold C, Watts S. Brody's human pharmacology. Antiarrhythmic drugs. 5th ed. Mosby, Inc; 2010. p. 242–54.

Algorithmic Approach to Pediatric ECG Interpretation

10

Ra-id Abdulla

This chapter provides an analytical approach to electrocardiogram (ECG) reading. The ECG findings of various lesions and disease processes are well described in the previous chapters of this book. This chapter provides a practical approach of how to analyze normal and abnormal findings of an ECG using a methodological approach through an algorithmic process which enables the formulation of a differential diagnosis.

A stepwise process in interpreting a 12 lead ECG is a must. Table 10.1 lists the various steps which must be performed. Although the order of these steps is not essential, sticking to any one particular order is a good habit to have so as to avoid overlooking an essential detail buried among other more prominent abnormal findings. A good example of this is overlooking an atrial abnormality such as right or left atrial enlargement when overwhelmed by a strikingly abnormal rhythm such as frequent premature ventricular contractions. Therefore, always follow an order.

Patient's Name

This step may seem too obvious to state, unfortunately though it is frequently ignored when reading a stack of ECGs. Knowing who the patient is, any previously established cardiac diagnoses and most importantly why the ECG was ordered can put in focus what is sought from this test. Comparing an ECG to previous ones is very helpful. A good example of the above is a patient with tachyarrhythmia. A wide QRS complex tachycardia may suggest ventricular

tachycardia; however, comparison with a previous ECG while in normal sinus rhythm which shows a right bundle branch block QRS pattern, similar to the QRS appearance when in tachyarrhythmia, should allow the conclusion that the tachyarrhythmia is actually of a more benign supraventricular origin. Reading print ECG is becoming less frequent as there is more reliance on electronic medical records; this allows comparison to previous ECGs which significantly adds to accuracy of diagnosis.

Patient's Age

As in most aspects of pediatric care, data can only be interpreted according to a child's age. What is considered normal for a newborn is likely to be abnormal in an adolescent. Therefore, noting patient's age is an essential initial step in assessing an ECG. Heart rate, PR and QRS intervals, QRS axis, and dominance of right versus left ventricular forces are all age dependent. A normal neonatal ECG, without the age being known, can be mistakenly read as sinus tachycardia, right axis deviation, and right ventricular hypertrophy with strain pattern. Table 10.1 in the Appendix section provides the normal values for each age group.

Patient's Sex

There is a limited role for patient's sex in interpreting an ECG; however, it is potentially important. Teenage boys may exhibit generous left ventricular forces through prominent R waves in left chest leads suggestive of left ventricular hypertrophy. This is also noted in athletes. When considering age and sex of patient, this may be considered to be within normal limits. In addition, QTc intervals are typically 10 msec longer in females.

10

R. Abdulla, MD
Pediatric Cardiology, Rush University Medical Center,
Chicago, IL, USA
e-mail: rabdulla@rush.edu

© Springer International Publishing Switzerland 2016
R. Abdulla et al. (eds.), *Pediatric Electrocardiography: An Algorithmic Approach to Interpretation*,
DOI 10.1007/978-3-319-26258-1_10

Table 10.1 Initial steps in assessing a 12-lead ECG

Patient's name
Patient's age
Patient's sex
Standardization of ECG
Heart rate
P wave axis
P wave height/width
P-QRS relationship
QRS axis
QRS duration
QRS amplitude
QT and QTc
ST segment
T waves
Prominent U wave
Right ventricle forces
Left ventricle forces

Standardization of ECG

Noting ECG standardization is an essential initial step when reading an ECG. Failing to note this will result in wrong interpretation. Please refer to Chap. 1 for details on this issue. Two types of standardization should be noted: voltage and paper speed standardizations. Voltage standardization is expressed in mV per millimeter (height of one small square). Full (or normal) standardization is 1 mV per 10 mm. When the QRS complexes are too tall or too deep, QRS complexes of different leads will overlap and make it difficult to measure an R's height or an S's depth. Therefore, ECG machines are equipped with ½ and ¼ standardization to minimize QRS complex overlap. Some ECG machines automatically flip to half standardization whenever an overlap is detected; therefore, noting the standardization is crucial. Heights and depths must be adjusted to the standardization as described in Chap. 1.

Paper speed standardization on the other hand must be activated manually. This is employed whenever there is tachyarrhythmia and the P waves are not clearly visualized. Doubling the speed of paper will require that all intervals be divided by 2 when calculating heart rate or measuring any periods.

Heart Rate

Sinus bradycardia, tachycardia, and arrhythmia may be encountered in a number of conditions. For bradyarrhythmia and tachyarrhythmia other than sinus, please refer to the section on interpretation of cardiac arrhythmia at the end of this chapter.

Bradycardia:
- Hypercalcemia
- Digoxin
- Quinidine/procainamide (toxic levels)
- Hypothyroidism
- Anorexia and malnutrition

Tachycardia:
- Fever
- Anxiety
- Sympathomimetic agents such as decongestants and asthma bronchodilators
- Thyrotoxicosis or excessive thyroid medications
- High catecholamine production such as with pheochromocytoma and other tumors

P Wave Axis

P wave axis 0–90°:
- A normal P wave axis is around 60° or positive P wave in leads I and aVL. Abnormal P wave axis reflects abnormal sinus node location or a cardiac pacemaker other than the sinus node.
- A normal P wave axis cannot rule out an ectopic atrial rhythm close to the sinus node (high right atrium). This may be suspected if the heart rate is fixed and/or fast (ectopic atrial tachycardia)

P wave axis 90–180°:
- Abnormal lead connection
- A high left atrial origin of P wave:
  - Left-sided sinus node, such as with:
    - Situs inversus.
    - Right isomerism; through this case, two different P waves may be present.

P wave axis 180–270°:
- Ectopic low left atrium

P wave axis 270–0°:
- Ectopic low right atrium

P Wave Height/Width

A normal P wave is 2 mm in height and 0.8–0.12 s in duration (2–3 small squares) depending upon age (younger children 2, older children and adults 3 small squares).

Tall P waves:
- Right atrial enlargement
- Increase intracranial pressure

Wide P waves:
- Left atrial enlargement

Low-voltage P wave:
- Hyperkalemia (severe)

Absent P wave:
- Hyperkalemia (severe)
- Associated with tachyarrhythmia:
  - Supraventricular tachycardia (SVT)
  - Junctional ectopic tachycardia (JET)
  - Ventricular tachycardia
- Junctional rhythm
- Ventricular rhythm
- Variable appearance of P waves: sick sinus rhythm or multifocal atrial tachycardia

PR Interval

Prolonged PR interval:
- Hypermagnesemia
- Digoxin
- Beta-blocking agents (class II)
- Amiodarone/sotalol (class III)

Short PR interval:
- Preexcitation, such as Wolff-Parkinson-White syndrome
- Class IA antiarrhythmic agents such as quinidine and procainamide
- Class IB antiarrhythmic agents such as lidocaine

PR depression:
- Pericarditis

P-QRS Relationship

AV block: AV block is of various types (see below section "Algorithmic approach to cardiac rhythm"). Most cases are idiopathic; occasionally, a cause could be detected, and this may include:

- Congenital heart disease, such as l-TGA and others
- Autoimmune disease, including maternal disease and in utero AV block
- Postoperative complication
- Post per-catheter septal occluding device
- Hyperkalemia
- Hypomagnesemia
- Digoxin
- Beta-blocking agents (class II)
- Amiodarone/sotalol (class III)

- Verapamil/diltiazem (class IV)
- Tricyclic antidepressants

QRS Axis

QRS axis 0–90°:
- Normal in all ages except neonates
- Left axis deviation in neonates:
  - LVH
  - Hypoplastic right ventricle

QRS axis 90–180°:
- Normal in neonates, infants, and young children
- Right axis deviation in adolescents and adults

QRS axis 180–270°:
- Right axis deviation:
  - Right ventricular hypertrophy
  - Hypoplastic left ventricle
- Superior axis deviation:
  - Atrioventricular canal defect
  - Heterotaxy
  - Single ventricle
  - Tricuspid atresia

QRS axis 270–0°:
- Normal in adults when within 0-30° Left axis deviation:
  - Left ventricular hypertrophy

QRS Duration

Prolonged:
- Bundle branch block; most common observation is with postsurgical closure of VSD.
- Preexcitation due to bypass tract.
- Hyperkalemia (nonspecific ventricular conduction delay or bundle branch block).
- Hypermagnesemia.
- Quinidine/procainamide.

QRS Amplitude

Diminished:
- Hypothyroidism
- Chagas disease
- Pericardial effusion
- Myocarditis

Increased:
- Chamber hypertrophy: RVH if in right chest leads (V1, 2) and LVH in left chest leads (V5, 6)

- If increased voltage noted in ectopic beats only: premature ventricular contractions

QT and QTc

Prolonged QT:
- Hypocalcemia
- Hypomagnesemia
- Hypoxia/acidosis
- Diphtheria
- Increase intracranial pressure
- Quinidine/procainamide
- Selective serotonin reuptake inhibitors (SSRIs)
- Antipsychotics

Shorten QT:
- Digoxin
- Lidocaine (and other class IB)
- Beta-blocking agents (class II)
- Halothane

ST Segment

Depression:
- Hypokalemia
- Anthracyclines
- Associated with elevated ST segment in other leads

Elevation:
- Benign if in one lead only
- Early repolarization
- Ischemia
- Pericarditis
- Myocarditis

Shortened:
- Hypercalcemia
- Hypermagnesemia

T Waves

Tall T wave:
- Hyperkalemia
- Diminished T wave amplitude:
- Hypokalemia
- Hypomagnesemia

Inverted:
- Ischemia
- Strain
- Myocarditis

Prominent U Wave

- Hypokalemia
- Hypomagnesemia

Right Ventricular Forces

Increased:
- Normal newborn RV dominance (R wave amplitude should not exceed what is expected for age)
- RVH
- Abnormal cardiac position within the chest:
  - Dextrocardia
  - Dextroposition
- Ventricular inversion:
  - Isolated ventricular inversion
  - l-TGA

Decreased:
- RV hypoplasia

Left Ventricular Forces

Increased:
- Left ventricular hypertrophy
- Athlete
- Thin chest wall
- Teenage, particularly boys and African-American ethnicity

Decreased:
- LV hypoplasia
- Abnormal cardiac position within the chest:
  - Dextrocardia
  - Dextroposition
- Ventricular inversion:
  - Isolated
  - l-TGA

Diagnosis Through Noting Combination of ECG Findings

Diagnosis may be reached through observing a combination of abnormal ECG findings. Cardiac lesions, congenital and acquired, typically affect more than one cardiac chamber. Through analytical thinking of the combination of abnormal ECG findings, a better understanding of abnormal hemodynamics can be achieved resulting in a list of potential diagnoses.

See Table 10.2 for abbreviations.

Table 10.2 Common ECG abbreviations

Abbreviation	Term
LAD	Left axis deviation
LAE	Left atrial enlargement
LVH	Left ventricular hypertrophy
RAD	Right axis deviation
RAE	Right atrial enlargement
RVH	Right ventricular hypertrophy
SAD	Superior axis deviation

RAE and RVH

This suggests increase volume or pressure load of the right heart, such as with:

- Atrial septal defect
- Partial anomalous pulmonary venous drainage
- Systemic arteriovenous malformation
- Tricuspid regurgitation
- Pulmonary stenosis and/or regurgitation and right heart failure
- Severe branch pulmonary artery stenosis
- Pulmonary hypertension

RAE, RVH, and RAD

This is consistent with volume or pressure overload of the right heart; this is similar to the differential diagnosis list of RAE and RVH.

RAE, RVH, and LAD

This is uncommon; it suggests one or more of the lesions listed under RAE and RVH associated with one of the following:

- Left bundle branch block
- Paced ventricular rhythm
- Ventricular inversion
- Pectus excavatum

LAE and LVH

This suggests volume and/or pressure overload of the left heart, such as with:

- Patent ductus arteriosus
- Mitral regurgitation
- Aortic regurgitation or stenosis and left heart failure
- Coarctation of the aorta (severe/chronic) and left heart failure

- Systemic hypertension (severe/chronic)

RAE and LAE

This entails dual pathology, such as:

- ASD with mitral stenosis (valvar or supravalvar)
- ASD with mitral regurgitation
- ASD with left heart failure for any reason

RVH and LVH

This is usually due to volume overload of both ventricles such as with:

- Ventricular septal defect, particularly with atrioventricular canal defect which may be associated with regurgitation of the atrioventricular valve, further increasing volume overload.
- Polyvalvular disease causing tricuspid and mitral regurgitation.
- Combination of pulmonary and aortic regurgitation due to:
  - Polyvalvular disease affecting pulmonary and aortic valves
  - Systemic disease, such as bacterial endocarditis affecting both pulmonary and aortic valves
  - Ross procedure with neo-aortic valve dilation leading to regurgitation, as well as regurgitation of the implanted pulmonary homograft
  - Repair of truncus arteriosus associated with regurgitation of truncal (neo-aortic) valve regurgitation and regurgitation of the implanted pulmonary homograft

Another possibility, though less common, is increase pressure load for both right and left ventricles:

- Williams disease: arterial stenosis leads to a wide spectrum of pulmonary and systemic arterial stenoses.

RAE, LAE, RVH, and LVH

Enlargement and hypertrophy of all cardiac chambers may be noted in:

- Severe anemia of any type resulting in expanded blood volume which overloads all cardiac chambers
- Left heart failure due to any cause which eventually leads to pulmonary hypertension which leads to right heart failure
- Severe AV valve regurgitation in patients with unrepaired AV canal defect

RAE, LAE, and RVH

Volume overload of the right heart due to a left ventricle to right atrium fistula will overload the right atrium and right ventricle. The resulting increase in pulmonary blood flow will overload the left atrium resulting in this unusual combination of ECG findings. This fistula is seen in:

- Gerbode defect, a congenital defect in the membranous portion of the ventricular septum where the left ventricle is separated from the right atrium by the membranous ventricular septum due to the slight apical displacement of the origin of the tricuspid valve septal leaflet. Defect in this region will connect the left ventricle to the right atrium, rather than the right ventricle.

- A similar type of shunt can be noted to that of Gerbode defect in patients with VSD bad defective tricuspid valve leading to left ventricle to right atrium shunt through the VSD and defective tricuspid valve.
- Acquired left ventricle to right atrium is seen in cases of prosthetic valve placement with resulting communication with the right atrium, similar to Gerbode defect or due to bacterial endocarditis of that portion of the ventricular septum or post atrioventricular septal defect surgical repair.

Algorithmic Approach to Cardiac Rhythm

Regular rhythm	Slow rate	Normal QRS	Normal P wave	Sinus bradycardia 2° AVB 3° AVB
			Abnormal P wave	Escape atrial rhythm
			No P wave	Escape junctional rhythm
		Wide QRS	Normal P wave	Sinus bradycardia + BBB 2° AVB + BBB 3° AVB + BBB
			Abnormal P wave	Escape atrial rhythm + BBB
			No P wave	Escape junctional rhythm + BBB
	Normal rate	Normal QRS	Normal P wave	Normal sinus rhythm
			Abnormal P wave	Atrial flutter with high degree AV block
			No P wave	Accelerated junctional rhythm
		Wide QRS	Normal P wave	NSR + BBB
			Abnormal P wave	Atrial flutter with AV block + BBB
			No P wave	Accelerated junctional rhythm + BBB
	Fast rate	Normal QRS	Normal P wave	Sinus tachycardia
			Abnormal P wave	Atrial flutter Ectopic atrial tachycardia
			No P wave	Supraventricular tachycardia Junctional ectopic tachycardia
		Wide QRS	Normal P wave	Sinus tachycardia + BBB
			Abnormal P wave	Atrial flutter + BBB Ectopic atrial tachycardia + BBB
			No P wave	Ventricular tachycardia
Irregular rhythm	Slow rate		2° AVB with variable conduction	
	Normal rate		Premature atrial contraction Premature ventricular contraction	
	Fast rate		Atrial fibrillation Atrial flutter with variable conduction Ventricular tachycardia Ventricular fibrillation	

Appendix

Table 1 Normal values for ECG parameters by age

Age	Heart rate (bpm)	QRS axis (degrees)	PR interval (ms)	QRS interval (ms)	R in V1 (mm)	R in V2 (mm)	S in V1 (mm)	R in V5 (mm)	R in V6 (mm)	S in V6 (mm)
1st week	90–160	60–180	80–150	30–80	5–26	5–30	0–23	1–20	0–12	0–10
1–3 weeks	100–180	45–160	80–150	30–80	3–21	8–29	0–16	1–23	2–16	0–10
1–2 months	120–180	30–135	80–150	30–80	3–18	8–30	0–15	10–33	5–21	0–10
3–5 months	105–185	0–135	80–150	30–80	3–20	10–31	0–15	10–34	6–22	0–10
6–11 months	110–170	0–135	70–160	30–80	2–20	12–31	0.5–20	10–31	6–23	0–7
1–2 years	90–165	0–110	80–160	30–80	2–18	7–31	0.5–21	10–33	6–23	0–7
3–4 years	70–140	0–110	90–170	40–80	1–18	6–27	0.5–21	12–38	4–24	0–5
5–7 years	65–140	0–110	90–170	40–80	0.5–14	5–25	0.5–24	15–38	4–26	0–4
8–11 years	60–130	−15–110	90–170	40–90	0–14	3–20	0.5–25	15–39	4–25	0–4
12–15 years	65–130	−15–110	90–170	40–90	0–14	3–18	0.5–21	8–35	4–25	0–4
>16 years	50–120	−15–110	90–170	40–100	0–14	3–18	0.5–23	8–35	4–21	0–4

bpm beats per minute

Table 2 PR interval by heart rate

Heart rate (bpm)	PR interval (ms)
>180	90–110
160–180	100–120
140–160	90–140
120–140	100–150
100–120	100–160
80–100	100–170
60–80	150–180
<60	160–190

bpm beats per minute

© Springer International Publishing Switzerland 2016
R. Abdulla et al. (eds.), *Pediatric Electrocardiography: An Algorithmic Approach to Interpretation*,
DOI 10.1007/978-3-319-26258-1

Table 3 Calculated QTc using observed QT and heart rate (HR)

Heart rate (bpm)	Measured QT interval (s)						
	0.20	0.25	0.30	0.35	0.40	0.45	0.50
50	0.18	0.23	0.27	0.32	0.37	0.41	0.46
52	0.19	0.23	0.28	0.32	0.37	0.42	0.46
54	0.19	0.23	0.28	0.33	0.38	0.42	0.47
56	0.19	0.24	0.29	0.34	0.38	0.43	0.48
58	0.20	0.24	0.29	0.34	0.39	0.44	0.49
60	0.20	0.25	0.30	0.35	0.40	0.45	0.50
63	0.21	0.25	0.31	0.36	0.41	0.46	0.51
66	0.21	0.26	0.31	0.36	0.42	0.47	0.52
68	0.22	0.26	0.32	0.37	0.43	0.48	0.53
71	0.22	0.27	0.33	0.38	0.44	0.49	0.55
75	0.23	0.27	0.34	0.39	0.45	0.51	0.56
79	0.24	0.28	0.34	0.40	0.46	0.52	0.57
83	0.24	0.29	0.35	0.41	0.47	0.53	0.69
88	0.25	0.29	0.36	0.43	0.49	0.55	0.61
94	0.26	0.30	0.38	0.44	0.50	0.56	0.63
100	0.27	0.31	0.39	0.45	0.52	0.58	0.65
107	0.28	0.32	0.40	0.47	0.53	0.60	0.67
115	0.28	0.35	0.42	0.49	0.55	0.63	0.69
125	0.29	0.36	0.43	0.51	0.58	0.65	0.72
136	0.30	0.38	0.45	0.53	0.60	0.68	0.75
150	0.32	0.40	0.47	0.56	0.63	0.71	0.79

Example: a patient with a measured QT of 0.30 s and a heart rate of 75 bpm has a c QTc of 0.34 s

bpm beats per minute

Index

© Springer International Publishing Switzerland 2016
R. Abdulla et al. (eds.), *Pediatric Electrocardiography: An Algorithmic Approach to Interpretation*,
DOI 10.1007/978-3-319-26258-1